BEAT ANXIETY & PANIC ATTACKS (2 IN 1)

OVERCOMING YOUR SOCIAL ANXIETY (IN RELATIONSHIPS) & DEPRESSION NATURALLY USING THERAPY (CBT & DBT & ACT), MEDITATIONS & HEALTHY LIVING

WESTLEY ARMSTRONG

D

DEVON HOUSE
PRESS

CONTENTS

Part III
MAKING THE NEW LIFESTYLE LAST

INTRODUCTION

We live in a society that conditions us into the belief that certain feelings are bad and that being positive and happy all the time is the way things should be. So, if you're a kid who doesn't fit that description (like me) or if something happens along your journey and you realize you're not happy all the time, all of a sudden, there's cause for alarm. When we feel anxious, stressed, overwhelmed, or nervous, we often get mad at ourselves for having these feelings because we believe it's wrong to feel that way. Usually, we'll tend to avoid the people, situations, or places that stir up these feelings as children. But as we grow up, we realize these feelings are EVERYWHERE! So, where does that leave us?

Transitioning into adulthood in our generation is unlike anything our parents and great-grandparents experienced. Disruptive change is real. Our world is changing in ways none of us expected, much less feel equipped to handle.

Even if you spend years getting a formal education and putting your-self into debt for a college degree, that still doesn't guarantee you'll have a great and happy life. Previous generations seemed to have a much easier time as life was slower, more pre-determined, and the economy less volatile than today. So, it was easier to predict the kind of life that awaited you if you did everything by the books. Today, it's a different story. Is it any wonder mental health has become such a hot issue in our society?

And it doesn't just affect adults. Even young teens and pre-teens find themselves trapped in a mind and body that doesn't function opti-mally. All doctors can say is "try not to worry so much "... I find that to be one of the most irritating lines anyone could tell me. And I've heard that statement far too many times for my taste. And you prob-ably picked up this book because you're fed up with something.

Perhaps you're sick and tired of going through life feeling trapped and unable to function like the friends you grew up with. You might have realized that your current lifestyle isn't sustainable. The fact that you can barely keep friends or that you'd rather drive for 12 hours than catch a thirty-minute flight because you can't handle flying isn't going to make life more comfortable as you grow older.

And given how important public speaking, social gatherings, and networking has become for a successful career, it's time to make some changes. But maybe for you, it's not even about being social. Perhaps your problem is far worse, and you're sick and tired of relying on medication and changing therapists because nothing works. Each year as the economy shifts and your debts increase, you might be feeling like you're about to lose your mind.

I don't want to come across like a know-it-all. I am aware that your story might be entirely different from the various scenarios I just shared, but here's the thing. You were attracted to this guide because, for one reason or another, you're tired of falling victim to the torturous reign of anxiety and panic attacks.

When anxiety or panic strikes for the first time, all you want to do is escape that experience. Suppose it's linked to a particular location or person. In that case, the natural inclination is to avoid that place or person altogether, especially when it happens the third or fourth time. As the problem keeps recurring in different places, you start wondering if it might be caused by you. Perhaps you are to blame. But it feels hard to own that you need help. Ultimately, there comes a day when it's you, on your couch, in the shower, or lying in bed, unable to fall asleep. For no apparent reason, full-blown anxiety attacks out of the blue, and you know for a fact that you need serious help!

Unfortunately for many of us, it takes a while before it dawns on us that this horrible experience is actually shadowing us because it's coming from within. The day you realize that is probably one of the worst days in your life because suddenly you feel completely power-less and unable to escape this invisible prison.

I've been there too.

At the age of eleven, I had my first panic attack. I couldn't figure out what was happening, but it was an overwhelming feeling that I had no control over. I honestly thought my heart was going to burst out of my chest. I tried to hide my symptoms because we were at a dinner gathering with my parents, and I didn't want to become the center of attention.

I felt dizzy, my vision was blurry, and I think for a moment there, I may have lost consciousness. Lucky for me, I was able to run outside to the backyard and just lie on the grass until I felt a little better. If I'd had my way, I would have run all the way home that evening. But I had to contain myself to avoid annoying and embarrassing my parents. Besides, what would everyone think of me? Wouldn't they call me weak? I didn't want to put myself through that kind of shame. So, I sucked it up, and it seemed to work for a while. The following months seemed fine until another event triggered my anxiety. This time, it was more potent and impossible to hide. My parents were hosting a Christmas dinner with friends and family. I had been taking piano lessons for about a year, and I wasn't too bad but nowhere ready to perform for anyone. Unfortunately, my folks saw this as an opportunity to show off their son's talents. They told everyone I was going to perform something. It was the most horrifying moment when they announced it at the dinner table. Everyone saw me as the shy kid who barely speaks, but they were eager to hear me play. I wanted the earth to open up and swallow me whole.

By the time we got to the actual performance, I was sweating, feeling nauseous, dizzy, and almost about to faint. I recall my dad sitting down and playing a quick tune to prime the audience and encourage me, then he gestured for me to join him and play. I stood up and started walking toward him, then at some point, my body froze, turned around, and ran upstairs to my room almost at its own will. I barely made it to my bed. Lying in bed, I had a full-blown panic attack which caused my mom to freak out and rush me to the hospital. In the months and years that followed, these overwhelming feelings came back sporadically. By eighteen, I seemed to hit rock bottom. I had panic attacks almost everywhere I went. My social life went down to zero. I had to quit practically every hobby I had as a kid, and the thought of growing up into a man with a career while feeling as I did almost drove me mad. I just knew I couldn't handle life as it was. I'll spare you the agonizing details of having to go through life thinking that I would never have an active and fully functional life. Doctors could never find anything wrong with me, but I knew something wasn't right. The medication I was prescribed didn't seem to solve the problem, but at least it helped me cope. So, trust me, I am well aware of how debilitating anxiety disorders can be. The main reason for creating the resources that I've built over the years for overcoming anxiety and panic is because I got to a point in my life where I'd had enough. I was sick and tired of being a victim and feeling trapped. I needed a way out.

After years of darkness and feeling trapped in a nightmarish tunnel, I finally found a way out. The documentation of techniques and solutions that I used to heal and then test others with successful outcomes is what you hold in your hand. You will be presented with proven knowledge, methods, techniques, and options for therapy programs that do not involve any use of medication.

I've seen people transform their lives when they and those around them had already lost all hope. These people believed they were doomed to live with anxiety disorders forever and thought the best case scenario was getting coping strategies that brought some temporary relief. Luckily, they were wrong. You'll read some of those triumphant stories throughout the book. Understand that I'm not suggesting this will work for every single person out there suffering from anxiety and panic disorder. However, I believe that if you are committed to this process and if you find resonance in my holistic approach to healing, you can step out of powerlessness and into your new lifestyle.

Think of this as a guidebook that will give you useful and easy to apply solutions to overcome your anxiety and panic attacks so that you can finally live the happy life you deserve. Excited? Good. Let's dive in.

I

FUNDAMENTALS ON ANXIETY, PANIC ATTACKS, AND STARTING YOUR ROAD TO OVERCOMING IT

WHY OUR NATURAL STATE IS PEACE & HAPPINESS, DESPITE THE MAJORITY OF US DRIFTING SO FAR FROM IT, AND HOW TO GET MORE IN TOUCH WITH YOUR NATURAL BEING!

What does Happiness mean to you? How do you define Peace?

I f you were to seek dictionary definitions of these two terms, you would have an intellectual earful of concepts that sound good but do nothing to transform your life.

It is futile to use someone else's definition of happiness and peace because that doesn't get you any closer to having it in your life. Most personal development students talk about peace and happiness. Many spiritual gurus teach about inner peace and happiness, but that still doesn't help the masses. There's a massive difference between knowing about something and experiencing it.

Have you ever watched a good deep-sea documentary where you saw the ocean's tide crashing against the shore with so much drama and intensity? Then as the camera ventures, a few meters down, you see a tranquil new world filled with all kinds of beautiful creatures, moving at their own pace, wholly unfazed by the action up above? This is fantastic imagery to help you understand what peace and happiness are like. You see, most of us tend to live on the surface of the waves where there's a lot of turbulence and wildness. The problem is that's the only way we know to live life. We fail to realize that there's another deeper level within us where everything is calm, blissful, and steady. This level of relaxed awareness is actually within each of us. What we need is access.

For that reason, I don't want to shove down your throat intellectual definitions that will do nothing more than entertain you for a minute. Instead, I want to invite you to reflect as you read this section of the book. Bring to mind any moments in your life, either through observation or direct experience, where you have felt happy. Think also to moments when you have felt in complete peace. That was you catching a glimpse of peace and happiness. It was you catching a whiff of your true nature. No matter how fleeting and temporary that moment, if you can bring it to mind, you can begin this process of understanding what peace and happiness mean.

Have you ever taken a moment to observe young babies playing in a park or by the beach? What's one word that comes to mind when most people think of such a scenario? I'd contend that majority would say happy, *i.e., children always look so glad.* Even when they get upset over a broken toy or falling down while running after a bunny in the yard, they quickly default back to that state we'd often refer to as happiness.

Now, let's try another scenario. You're stuck in line at the pharmacy, and the contents of your bag spills on the floor just as your phone starts ringing! I'm guessing the first impulse would probably be a stream of four-letter words that no one should hear. And even if you manage to suppress that urge to unleash your anger and frustration, we know that negative outburst isn't too far from your default setting. After all, anxiety and panic have never been associated with peace and happiness. So, what gives?

Is this happiness thing something that only young babies and the chosen few can enjoy?

The truth is actually going to feel outrageous for you. Especially if you've spent the last couple of years in deep emotional winter. Happiness is our natural state of being. Peace in mind, body, and spirit is how you were meant to experience this journey of being human!

Peace and happiness are our natural state, and most of us don't know it.

Bet you've heard of expensive beach yoga retreats that people invest a fortune in just to catch a glimpse of what peace and happiness might be like. The driving motive behind this desire to seek out happiness is actually good. Where most of us go wrong is that we assume it is something that doesn't belong to us and that we need to work hard to attain. We see it in the same light as hitting a target at work, and that's where we often fall off track. Peace and happiness are already part of our DNA. It's who we are. But even the most beautiful rose garden, when neglected and left unkempt, will develop weeds. And the weeds will choke all the beauty and cause one to wonder if there were ever rose bushes in that garden.

What I'm trying to put across is that your natural state of happiness and peace was impeded for one reason or another. The work then isn't to get something you don't have but instead restore yourself to that original natural state before your weeds took over and messed with your mind and life. When we look for circumstances to help us achieve inner peace, we end up further away from our source of happiness and only aggravate the anxiety that ails us.

HAPPINESS FROM A SCIENTIFIC APPROACH

The study of happiness has grown dramatically in the last three decades. One of the most common questions happiness investigators examine is this: How happy are people in general? In a 2007 survey, Gallup found that 52% of U.S adults who took the survey reported they were very happy. 8 out of 10 indicated they were very satisfied with their lives. Another poll done in 2013 revealed that happiness was trending downward. Only a third of the participants of this recent survey reported being very happy. Certain groups, including minorities, recent college graduates, and the disabled, revealed a decline in their happiness levels. I can only imagine what the polls would show now after being hit by a 2021 global pandemic, a crazy Trump era, and a massive unemployment rate in 2020.

It is Suffice to say, happiness is something many people are trying to understand. Few have successfully managed to get it. Happiness investigators looking to discover what makes people happy were searching to see if money, attractiveness, material possessions, satisfying relationships, or a rewarding occupation played a role in securing happiness in an individual. They still don't know with certainty. What they speculate is that age is related to happiness. Life satisfaction usually increases the older people get, but there does not appear to be gender differences in happiness (Diener, Suh, Lucas & Smith, 1999).

HOW DID WE DRIFT FAR FROM OUR NATURAL STATE?

This is a question that has no shortage of answers. You just need to look around. The addiction to technology we're all guilty of. Uncertainty of everything, including climate change, wars, sexual predators, government officials who are sometimes unfit to become heads of states, random shootings, pandemics, and the list goes on and on. I mean, unless you live in a cave, there's enough news reaching you that makes even a mentally healthy person anxious. For those already struggling with mental health disorders, especially anxiety and panic, things only get worse. It's hard not to feel angry, sad, powerless, and basically defeated by life. That is the opposite of joy and peace.

There's also plenty of research conducted by social psychologists reported in the Greater Good Magazine that suggests our happiness and peace of mind have been dwindling at incredible speeds since the 1950s, mainly due to our disconnection from nature. These studies, along with hundreds of others, point to the conclusion that we stand to benefit tremendously from nurturing a strong connection with nature. The more connected we are, the happier we are. The reverse is also true.

Some might think that this shift happened due to urbanization, but in fact, popular culture shows it has more to do with the lifestyle shift we made with the advent of technology that moved us further away from nature.

Take a personal inventory of how much time you spend watching sunsets, strolling on a park/beach, or sitting in a garden on Sunday afternoons. Now contrast that total time with the amount you spend indoors watching Netflix, on the couch, or in bed surfing the Internet or social media. You'll learn a thing or two about your current connection to the nature around you. And by that logic, the further away you feel from nature, the harder it will be to nurture the joy, power, and peace of mind you're seeking.

PANIC ATTACKS AND ANXIETY CAN OCCUR WHEN YOU DRIFT APART

After learning that your natural state is happiness and peace of mind, I hope you can already see that your anxiety issues are not meant to be with you forever. They exist because something went wrong and caused you to drift from your natural state of being. Before we can help you get back to your true self and heal the current issue, we need to understand what you're suffering from, the cause of it, and how to treat it.

Anxiety is a mental health problem that can take different forms. There is a normal level of stress that almost everyone experiences whenever there is real danger or cause for concern. For example, if you just lost your job, your brain would trigger those anxious feelings as a way to motivate you to solve the problem before next month's bills are due. That is not what this book is about. Our focus is on anxiety disorders which are a group of mental illnesses that cause constant overwhelm and fear. These excessive emotions make it difficult to function normally at work, school, home, and socially. To the degree your anxiety is left unchecked, to that degree, it will get worse. There are many types of anxiety, including generalized anxiety disorder, panic disorder, social anxiety disorder, phobia, separation anxiety, selective mutism, medication-induced anxiety, and so many others. This book's focus will remain on panic disorders, social anxiety, and general anxiety, but let's briefly define what each of the above-mentioned looks like.

- **Selective mutism:** This isn't a prevalent type of social anxiety, but some people suffer from it. Usually, it will be in young children and some teens who typically talk with their family but don't speak publicly.
- **Medication induced anxiety:** This occurs when a person uses a particular medication or even illegal drugs, which triggers anxiety symptoms. It can also happen if one withdraws from taking a specific medicine. For example, if you've been on anti-depressants for a long time and stop taking them, it might trigger anxiety.
- **Separation anxiety:** This form of anxiety is more common in your children, but you can also find it in adults. If you often feel anxious or fearful when a person you're close to leaves your sight or if you always worry that

something terrible may happen to your loved ones, then you're likely experiencing separation anxiety.

- **Phobias:** This isn't just about fearing a specific object or thing. It's more intense than that. The fear goes beyond what's appropriate, causing a severe biological reaction. For example, if you fear heights or flying, then being on a plane makes you sick, literally. Rock climbing even in a simulated closed room would cause you to faint or go into panic mode.
- **Panic disorder:** This type of anxiety is intense and will be our primary focus. It's when you get so fearful to the point of panic that you break into a sweat. Your heart pounds almost out of your chest, and you feel like you're having a heart attack. You might also get chest pains and start choking.
- **Generalized anxiety disorder:** This involves excessive unrealistic worry and tension with little or no reason.
- **Social anxiety disorder:** Often referred to as social phobia, people suffering from this are very self-conscious, constantly obsess about others judging them and often feel overwhelmed by negative emotions and worry. Being social is a great struggle, and they often withdraw from everyday social interactions.

A great question to ask would be, "what are some of the reasons I have drifted away from my natural state of being?

Instead of seeking external causes and reasons for your anxiety, it's time to look within. That's the only place you have control anyways. You cannot control people, the government, the economic markets, or the weather. So, does that mean you go through life forever helpless? Absolutely not. Instead, you want to become more aware of some of the things you might be doing that nurtures your anxiety. Here are a few common ways we tend to drift from our natural state.

#1: We worry about the future too much.

#2: Comparing yourself to others and how they do something can cause you to drift and block happiness.

#3: Getting too caught up in your head and over-thinking everything.

#4: Holding on to resentment, anger, or regret.

#5: Negative thoughts and emotions. Allowing negative emotions to consume your mind can eventually create a permanent state of anxiety. That's why it's imperative to learn how to observe, process, and control your emotions, so they don't rule your life.

#6: False interpretation and stories that create negative meanings, such as assuming people are criticizing, judging, or ridiculing you when they are not.

#7: Guilt and shame are big ones. Feeling ashamed for making a mistake or embarrassed that you've failed at something can set off a cycle of anxiety that blows up into something serious.

#8: Fear is by far the biggest emotion that creates anxiety and other mental health disorders. Suppose it becomes a permanent state of living. In that case, it can drive you into mental instability and completely block out peace and happiness in your life.

KEEP YOUR LINES OPEN, AND GET IN TOUCH WITH YOUR NATURAL BEING

When it comes to healing and recovering your natural state of being, there's no miracle required. You live in a universe that has limitless potential for joy built into the creation process. It doesn't matter how far you've drifted from that place of peace and real happiness. You can always find your way back. This book's contents will help you get in touch with your true nature once again so you can finally have the kind of life you always dreamed of. It begins with a deep understanding of your thoughts and a clear recognition of who you really are. Yes, there's plenty of external reasons in the world to trigger stress and worry. Still, peace and happiness should never be at the mercy of conditions.

If being happy was a matter of having a perfect, problem-free life without any challenges, this whole conquest would be futile. What you need to understand is that being happy and at peace is an inner game. It's not about changing the outside world or fighting against the wrong things. Instead, it's about choosing your personal peace and happiness. It's about finding ease and training your mind to practice thoughts of minimal resistance until it becomes your natural way of reacting to conditions. Eventually, you'll become the kind of person you've always wanted to be free of the "dis-ease" that stress brings to your body.

Are you ready to choose peace and Happiness?

THE 3 BIGGEST MYTHS ABOUT ANXIETY DEBUNKED!

L et get something cleared up now. Anxiety disorders are real and should be treated with the same urgency as any physical disorder. Anxiety disorders are common and pervasive in the U.S. It is estimated that nearly 40 million people in the United States experience an anxiety disorder in any given year. Still, there's a lot of stigma around anxiety, and it's time to set the record straight. So here are three myths we need to debunk.

ANXIETY ISN'T A REAL ILLNESS; IT'S ALL MADE UP!

Everyone gets a little anxious from time to time. Worry over landing a job, a case of nerves before a big test, feeling nervous before a first date, or difficulty sleeping after a traumatic event are all normal. But when excessive anxiety takes over and persists in interfering with your daily thoughts and activities, it's time to seek professional help.

There's nothing ordinary about recurring nightmares, flashbacks, panic attacks that seemingly come out of the blue, or avoiding social situations because you fear being judged, embarrassed, or humiliated. The worst thing you can do is assume you are weak or try to hide the symptoms. Instead, you need to get help because it won't just go away. You can't wish it away or ignore it any more than you can a heart attack or diabetes.

The only way to treat anxiety is with medication, therapy, meditation, and other healthy lifestyle changes. So, don't let anyone make you feel like it's all in your head; it isn't!

PEOPLE WHO HAVE ANXIETY ARE WEAK, IT'S A CHOICE THAT THESE PEOPLE CHOOSE TO HAVE

Some people assume that anxiety can be switched on and off. As though it's a personal choice, but that is so far from the truth. Others think it's a way of getting attention from the people in your life. This is totally false. The fact is anxiety affects your body, mind, and behavior. It's a condition that can affect people of all ages, in all walks of life. So, we need to discard this false perception that people with anxiety are weak or broken somehow. It's one of the key reasons most people struggle in silence (mostly men). There's no shame in suffering from this mental disorder. You should approach it the same way you would bronchitis or any other health condition.

ANXIETY CAN ONLY BE TREATED THROUGH MEDICATION

Many assume that the only treatment for anxiety is medication. But as you'll discover in this book, there are many ways to heal yourself. Nowadays, medicine is perhaps the least desirable because of the side effects that follow. Although there are many cases where medication is recommended, it has to be combined with something that can address the root issue. Usually, medicine only provides a temporary remedy and a sense of relief, but to cure anxiety, one must tackle the root problem.

The most effective treatment is a particular type of therapy known as Cognitive Behavioral Therapy (CBT), based on mindfulness and changing your thinking, attitudes, behavior, and beliefs.

DO YOU KNOW WHAT MAKES YOU AFRAID?

Fear is at the root of any anxiety disorder. But what is fear, and why are we so fearful? Lots of things make us afraid. Fear is a strong emotion that can quickly rule your mind and life if left unchecked. Our brains are naturally wired to trigger anxiety-based emotions when we feel threatened or in danger. This has proved extremely useful in our survival as a species, given how tiny we are and how wild and dangerous life used to be before civilization. I'm pretty sure fear was helpful when we were hunters and gatherers trying to avoid being eaten by lions and such. Today, however, it's a different story. We are experiencing high levels of fear when there's no real or imminent threat, but our brains can't seem to tell the difference. We can get really fearful of a person, place, an event that in no way threatens our life. But because our brains are accustomed to being in constant fear, we'll react the same way our ancestors did when facing a fatal situation. Our bodies seem to react in that same way even though we are not in any real danger. There are plenty of triggers for fear in everyday life. It may not be easy to figure out each and every trigger that causes your mind and body to shift into that stressful state, so what you need to do is better manage your emotions and how you react once fear kicks in. Once you understand your fears, it becomes easy to understand your anxiety.

WHAT MAKES YOU ANXIOUS EVEN WHEN THERE'S NO DANGER AROUND YOU

Health professionals usually use the term "anxious" to refer to persistent fear. So, anxiety and fear are inseparable. The primary feelings (whether you are very anxious or afraid) will likely be the same, and that's why you want to become aware of the things that make you fearful and anxious.

The experience of anxiety isn't restricted to the economically deprived or politically oppressed. Anyone can suffer from it. Many tend to deny their personal anxiety or at least its intensity, sometimes even to themselves for various reasons such as the fear of rejection, avoiding embarrassment, or a sense of pride. And while it is closely related to fear, they are not one and the same.

THE DIFFERENCE BETWEEN FEAR AND ANXIETY

It's essential to understand the difference between these two states so you can diagnose your current condition. Some have referred to anxiety as "fear spread out thin," which is because, at its root, anxiety is often fueled by some kind of fear. Fear is basically a survival mechanism. It's both the psychological and emotional response to a feeling of being in danger and is most concerned with self-preservation. Anxiety, on the other hand, is a warning signal of one's increasing inability to survive.

Did you know that not all forms of anxiety are considered harmful? Many psychologists believe that periodic mild stress and anxiety can assist in increasing performance and productivity. For certain individuals, alertness and motivation are enhanced, causing them to tap into their potential even more.

So, the topic of anxiety can feel quite controversial, much like stress. There seems to be amiable and pernicious anxiety, much like how we know there is good stress and bad stress or good cholesterol and bad cholesterol.

For example, suppose you ask an athlete, a performer, or anyone else about to embark on a life-changing event. In that case, they might disclose an experience of mild anxiety on their part. The science community seems to see this as something good. However, the threat to health occurs when sustained for long periods of time and begins to take a life of its own in your mind.

Here's something you need to know about anxiety: It's not a one-size-fits-all condition whereby we can assume that specific strategies will work for everyone across the board. For example, peace and quiet or eliminating stress from your life can be useful and great advice for one person but ineffective for another. For instance, I have a friend who feels that his anxiety worsens when in a quiet, slow-paced area. When he stays alone with his thoughts, he feels less productive, isolated, and abandoned, which doesn't really help. So, his strategies for managing and healing obviously cannot include an extended period of being locked up in a room for self-contemplation.

And with that, you should also note that there are basically two types of debilitating anxiety: simple and neurotic. As the name suggests, simple anxiety is temporary emotional tension often tied to life's struggles and pressures such as paying bills, passing a final exam, or an executive who is tasked with the burden of meeting an impossible quota.

Neurotic anxiety is emotional tension that has become ingrained into your behavior, making it part of your personality. Some neurosis includes obsessive-compulsive reaction, hysteria, chronic depression, among others. Untreated neurosis can, over time, develop into psychosis. However, this generally occurs for people with the heredity disposition of mental health problems.

Another odd thing about anxiety that I realized is that your triggers might change over time. For example, I used to feel extremely anxious whenever I was at the movie theater. One day, I noticed the tension had almost dissipated because I would go to the theater and not feel as bad as I once did. The alarm that would always go off in my head somehow got disarmed as my brain realized I wasn't in any real danger when I go out to see a movie. You might notice something similar in your life whereby some trigger that used to bother you suddenly dissipates. What you don't want is to have more triggers popping up. Your relationship with anxiety is likely going to evolve as you continue on this journey of healing.

IT IS WHAT IT IS

A panic attack is an intense wave of fear characterized by its unexpectedness and debilitating immobilizing intensity. When a panic attack hits, you can't breathe, your heart feels like it's going to burst right out of your chest, and you feel like you're about to die or go mad. Most of the time, the panic attack strikes out of the blue. There's no warning or prep time. Some people can notice the trigger just before it hits. Unfortunately, I was never one of those. My triggers just weren't clear enough, so I always missed them.

While science hasn't identified the definite cause of anxiety and panic attacks, enough evidence points to various things, including environmental factors, genetic predisposition, brain chemistry, medical history, traumatic life events, and prolonged exposure to stress. Use of or withdrawal from an illicit substance can also contribute to the development of anxiety.

THE MOST COMMON CAUSES OF ANXIETY

Genes

Specific gene variants may be associated with greater levels of stress and anxiety. We are all unique human beings with different biological make-up, so you might be one of those people who might experience greater levels of anxiety than your relatives or friends for no other reason but that it's embedded in your genetic code. You could receive the exact same news, and it would trigger something in you while it does nothing to the other person. For example, I can recall when my parents told my sibling and me that we would be spending a Saturday afternoon at a family friend's home for a summer party. I immediately started feeling nervous while my sibling didn't seem to care at all. Essentially, what happens for those like us is that the genes cause chemical imbalances in the brain, leading to heightened stress levels.

What to consider if your biology is prone to stress and anxiety:

A medical professional would be able to run a series of tests to determine this. They would advise the best treatment. Some psychiatrists might recommend medication. Proceed with caution if you choose to go for that option because most of the time, the side effects of relying on medication can be quite harmful in the long run. I suggest experimenting with combinations of other treatments first unless your case is extremely severe.

Health

Pent-up stress combined with a poor diet and physical inactivity can be a great source of anxiety disorder. Do you know that? When we mistreat our bodies, we often directly impact our mental state because our biology affects our psychology and vice versa. We mistreat our bodies when we indulge in stimulants to the point of addiction. When we eat the wrong food, engage in poor sleeping habits, and avoid keeping our bodies active.

If you're in the habit of skipping meals and binge-eating crappy, over-processed junk food, you're likely not having a balanced diet. Your body and brain are missing critical nutrition to maintain optimum functioning, which could very well cause or at least contribute to an anxiety disorder's build-up.

Think for a moment about the idea of having a gene that makes you prone to anxiety. If you're mistreating your body, then you're more likely to trigger anxiety and fall ill not because of the genes per se but because of the combination of these two factors. See how this works?

So, it's not enough to say that your friend Sally sleeps as little as you and eats crap all week yet never falls sick because you don't know Sally's biological disposition. So, you might both have the same health habits, but for you, it might lead to a mental health issue.

The same is true with lacking physical exercise because activities like running, swimming, playing sports, and working out in the gym are scientifically proven to benefit the body and brain. They help in stress management and the production of feel-good hormones. Physical exercise is a great way to channel hormones like adrenaline and corti-sol, avoiding stress and anxiety.

Unhealthy mental states

Two major tenuous mental states cause emotional disturbances: Guilt and egoism.

Guilt is the sense of personal wrongdoing and being liable for punishment. By its very nature, guilt always creates psychotic tension. It might be false or true, but the psychic experience and tension are similar and real to the person in either case. True guilt results from the transgression or rejection of either some authoritative or societally established law. For instance, if you steal something from someone, you may feel a sense of guilt.

On the other hand, false or imaginary guilt comes from the failure to conform to others' expectations or judgments. For instance, if you struggled to perform well in class, perhaps peers and even the teachers would mock your performance, leading to guilt. This guilt isn't justified, but it still causes damage. Many neuroses have guilt as their central component. Often the impetus underlying false guilt is the need to win someone's approval, the need to please, or to be accepted by others.

If, as you read this, something strikes a chord in you, there might be some unchecked guilt brewing. Ask yourself the following questions:

a. What kind of guilt am I experiencing or hiding?
b. Is it really justified?
c. What is the reason behind my guilt?
d. What would be the proper way to view this situation?

If you realize you're holding on to morally justified guilt, it's time to do something about it. If it's morally unjustified, then acknowledge it for what it is, recognize that it is harming your entire life, and resolve it once and for all. You might be inclined to think that anxiety is your enemy, but the truth is, guilt and any unresolved negative emotions are the real enemies that should be dealt with. Divorce yourself from any and all guilt.

Egoism is another troublesome mental state. Usually, people suffering from egoism are so preoccupied with their personal needs they have no idea they actually suffer from it. A common trait of being egoistic is anger. There are two fundamental dimensions to consider here: Arrogance comes from feeling superior, and inadequacy that comes from feeling inferior.

A superior disposition compels a person to obsessively strive for personal attention and secure others' praise. There's a lot of exaggeration involved and a strong need for recognition. Usually, such a person is insensitive, judgmental, and even merciless when it comes to others, making them potentially volatile. We can see a lot of this behavior in our current society, especially with celebrities and athletes. Some secondary mental states that accompany this dimension of egoism include bitterness, jealousy, resentment, and envy.

An inferior disposition is actually more prevalent in our world. Most people who suffer from anxiety actually suffer from an inferiority complex, causing them to socially withdraw and feel intimidated around people. Such a person feels unworthy of personal recognition and even love. I can speak of how this personally affected me. I used to feel like nothing I did was ever good enough or right. I felt like a complete failure in life.

For some people, this is developed from childhood, maybe because of how much parents criticized them or because they struggled to understand what was being taught in school. Usually, when a person suffers from an inferiority disposition, it's because they learn to dislike themselves and believe others don't like them either. The person never quite makes the grade, regardless of how hard they may try. Secondary mental states of an inferior disposition include discouragement, emptiness, depression, loneliness, insecurity, hatred, envy, and jealousy.

Sometimes anxiety is a result of a combination of multiple factors. So, the best advice is to run a simple self-analysis first to determine how many of the common symptoms are associated with anxiety and panic attacks and if they are persistent, seek professional assistance. This book will walk you through everything you need to know so you can take the necessary steps to heal. First, let's talk about the signs and symptoms of anxiety.

HOW SHOULD I KNOW: THE SIGNS AND SYMPTOMS

#1: Excessive worry

Worrying excessively is perhaps one of the most common symptoms of anxiety disorder. This isn't just concern over an upcoming exam or an overdue project you need to hand in. I'm talking about persistent worry that you can't escape from. It's almost like being choked by an invisible and inescapable force that only you can sense.

#2: Fatigue

Most people assume that anxiety disorder is always displayed as hyperactivity in an individual, but sometimes it can be the opposite. For some individuals, chronic fatigue is how anxiety expresses itself, especially after an anxiety attack. There might be a correlation between insomnia, muscle tension, hormonal imbalances, but this is not scientifically proven yet. Most of the time, when anxiety is coupled with depression, chronic fatigue is one of the symptoms you might notice.

#3: Severe Irritability

Do you find yourself often snapping at someone over something trivial? It could be a sign of anxiety disorder. This is another ubiquitous symptom of anxiety. According to a study with over six thousand adults, more than 90% of those diagnosed with generalized anxiety disorder said they often felt highly irritable during periods when their anxiety disorder was at its worst.

#4: Social distancing and avoidance

By this, I mean you avoid any social interactions and public places. If you tend to feel anxious or fearful about upcoming social situations or if you always worry that you'll be judged, ridiculed, or scrutinized by others, then you might be experiencing anxiety disorders. Approximately 12% of American adults suffer from an anxiety disorder at some point in their lives, so this is a fairly common condition. Most of the time, one can tell they suffer from it because they struggle to interact or socialize with others causing them to avoid parties, theaters, malls, and such places. While it's not always evident that someone is suffering from this condition as the person might just seem shy, snobby, or standoffish, it is a real disease that causes a lot of torment, extreme fear, and anxiety.

#5: Problems staying focused or concentrating on a task

A study including 157 children and teens diagnosed with GAD (generalized anxiety disorder) found that more than two-thirds of them had difficulty concentrating. Another study that assessed 175 adults also found that 90% reported having trouble concentrating. Those with severe anxiety issues seem to have the greatest level of difficulty maintaining their focus. Although the evidence isn't sufficient to claim poor concentration and decrease in performance with anxiety disorder, current results show that most people suffering from it will have issues concentrating.

#6: Restlessness

Anxiety in children and teens often shows up as restlessness. You will find yourself (or the person suffering from anxiety) always feeling "on edge." Doctors usually look for this symptom when trying to make a diagnosis. So, ask yourself how calm are you on a daily basis? Are you usually feeling the uncomfortable urge to move? Do you have trouble finding your calm zone most of the time?

#7: **Panic attacks**

Although panic attacks are a type of anxiety, they are also signs in and of themselves that you are suffering from an anxiety disorder. Panic attacks are incredibly intense and overwhelming. They usually reach their peak within 10 minutes and rarely last more than an hour. Sometimes they happen in isolation. They are often reoccurring and make it impossible for you to do things like driving for fear that you might have one and end up in an accident. Fear is always at the root of a panic attack. To diagnose a panic attack, look out for these signs:

a. Shortness of breath

b. A racing heart

c. Tingling numbness in the hands and fingers

d. Chest pains

e. Difficulty breathing

f. Overwhelming sensation of fear or impending doom or death

g. Feeling weak, faint, or dizzy

h. Nausea or upset stomach

i. Sweating

j. Choking feeling

k. Hot or cold flashes

BE CAREFUL, THERE ISN'T JUST ONE KIND.

There is a myriad of anxiety disorders that affect millions of people in the world. That's why you first need an accurate diagnosis of what you're suffering from so you can get proper treatment. If you haven't yet seen any particular symptom or type that matches what you're currently experiencing, here are some more common disorders to consider:

#1: Anxiety Attacks: With this disorder, you suddenly feel like you're about to pass out, go crazy, die, or lose control. You can also call it a panic disorder.

#2: Concerns about your appearance: This type of disorder causes you to feel like there's something abnormal or even grotesque about your appearance even though no one else sees that defect.

For example, imagine a wife who thinks, "*I think my hair is thinning.*" That creates anxiety and intrusive thoughts. She goes in front of the mirror, touches her head, and asks her husband, who responds, "*no honey, you've got beautiful, healthy hair.*" The woman feels better for about thirty seconds until another intrusive thought enters, "*he wasn't really listening to me. He never listens to me.*" Next thing you know, she's obsessing over baldness cures as she scours the internet for a solution.

This is a trivial example, but in some cases, it can be extreme to the point that a person refuses to undress or even enter into relationships because they believe they have a defect.

#3: Performance anxiety: Another type of anxiety that many struggles with is performing or competing in front of an audience. Some call this social anxiety disorder, but it can also be more intimate than just social performance. It can also include difficulty performing with an intimate partner.

#4: Agoraphobia: With this disorder, you're always afraid something terrible might happen if you're away from home. It could be the fear of having another panic attack and appearing distraught in public. You will notice that many people suffering from panic attacks also get agoraphobia.

#5: Shy bladder syndrome: With this condition, you have trouble using a public restroom. It's considered a form of social anxiety disorder.

#6: Post-traumatic stress disorder: This condition comes from a traumatic experience that you had in the past, which still has a firm emotional grip in your daily life. It could be child abuse, death of a loved one, rape, severe injury, or torture.

As you can see, there are many forms of anxiety. The more you can quickly identify with one, the higher the chances you're suffering from that type of mental disorder. Once you know what the problem is, finding the right solution becomes plausible. Don't feel pressured to label your condition and know that research is ongoing in the medical field, so this list is by far not extensive. If you don't find that you fit 100% in any particular disorder or that you have more than one ailing you, that's okay. This isn't something to criticize or feel ashamed about. You just need a starting point so you can gather the right resources and assistance to aid your healing.

CAN I CONTROL IT?

Often when we attempt to control our anxiety, we tend to make things worse. I think it's primarily because we approach it from a place of resistance. We get mad at ourselves for activating it and, in so doing, increase the intensity of the experience. Therefore, I want to suggest that your best efforts should be in self-acceptance and self-care strategies and not "controlling or eradicating feelings of uneasiness and anxiety." The more you can develop this mindset of focusing on constructive thinking and less on being in control all the time, the easier it will be to manage and recover from anxiety disorders.

One way of doing this is to learn healthy management strategies and to undergo treatment. In so doing, you can learn specific techniques that help you manage your condition. Many of the methods you will learn in the treatment options I will be sharing in the next chapter will help you practice things like progressive muscle relaxation, mindfulness meditation, deep breathing, and so much more. All of these will aid you in reducing anxiety symptoms. Through natural remedies, lifestyle changes, and the therapy options you will learn shortly, you can find a combination of solutions that enable you to permanently heal or at the very least manage anxiety.

4

HOW YOU CAN GET BACK TO ENJOYING YOUR LIFE & WHAT REALLY MATTERS TO YOU WITHOUT ANXIETY ALWAYS GETTING IN THE WAY

The cost of allowing anxiety to rule and ruin your life is profound and far-reaching. These effects fall into three basic categories: Physical, psycho-emotional, and social. Let's briefly look at each of these. Physically, you may continuously suffer from stomach issues, heart palpitations, headaches that won't go away, muscle cramps, and various inexplicable body aches and pains. Anxiety also increases the stress hormone cortisol, which raises blood pressure and contributes overtime to heart problems, stroke, kidney disease, and sexual dysfunction.

In a 2017 Lancet study using brain scans, they measured activity in an area called the amygdala, which mounts split-second responses to danger and encodes memories of frightening events. Greater activity in the amygdala correlated with a high risk for heart disease and stroke (sourced from Harvard Health Publishing - Anxiety: What it is, what to do). We know the amygdala is overactive for people suffering from anxiety, which might drive inflammation and plaque formation, leading to heart attacks and strokes.

When it comes to psycho-emotional disorders, we find that anxiety initially decreases performance by curtailing reasoning abilities, dulling imaginative thinking, and causing general discouragement. Anxiety disorders cause us to feel disoriented, discouraged, ashamed, and depression may then follow.

Your social life also takes a massive blow because extremely anxious people tend to avoid social contact even with familiar friends to cope with their situation. Social contact usually generates feelings of uncertainty, suspicion, and uneasiness. Overall, your quality of life suffers. It becomes impossible to have functional relationships or participate in activities that you previously enjoyed. With all this news of doom and gloom, it can be hard to see a way out of this nightmare experience. But I promise you it is possible when you realize this simple truth: You have the power to heal and transform your life.

IT STARTS WITH YOU

The road to overcoming anxiety and healing your life begins with a critical decision. You must choose to face your fear. The moment you become fed up with the current condition and feel like you've reached the end of the rope, that something must change is the turning point you will need to start your recovery. Once you choose to face your fear, the next step will be to accept the responsibility of knowing yourself and owning your ability to overcome this condition.

If you are at that point and you are ready to know more about yourself and the things that are triggering your anxiety, then you are primed to heal. With the right treatment and strategy, you will be on your path to recovery. But there are so many options for treatment. How do you know which to take? There's no right or wrong answer because it depends on your personality, the intensity of your anxiety, and what feels comfortable. Listen to your gut on this, and you won't go wrong. When it comes to therapy, my preferred options are Cognitive Behavioral Therapy, Dialectical Behavioral Therapy, and Acceptance Commitment Therapy. Let's discuss each in detail so you can identify which feels right.

GIVE COGNITIVE BEHAVIORAL THERAPY (CBT) A GO

Once you successfully diagnose your anxiety, it's essential to rule out the dominant cause of it. Suppose you're suffering from anxiety because of an underlying medical condition. In that case, you need a thorough physical exam to help resolve that physical malady first. But if your anxiety stems from the causes we mentioned earlier, and the doctors say physically you are in great shape, we can wholly focus on integrating proven treatments. Consider CBT, which many people claim is the most effective treatment for almost all forms of anxiety disorders. For this form of therapy two work, there are two critical aspects to consider. First, your willingness to change, and second is your relationship with your therapist.

What is CBT?

Cognitive-behavioral therapy is a form of short-term psychotherapy that focuses on your thoughts, beliefs, and attitudes and how that affects your feelings and behavior.

It can help your find new ways to behave by changing your thought patterns. It works on the basis that the way we think and interpret life's events often affects how we feel and behave. CBT centers on identifying and changing inaccurate or distorted thinking patterns, emotional responses, and behaviors. Cognitive-behavioral therapy techniques include cognitive restructuring and behavioral changes like reducing self-defeating behaviors and developing healthy habits.

It has been well researched, and studies conducted show that it can be powerful in treating a wide range of problems, including depression, anxiety disorders, insomnia, eating disorders, alcohol, and drug use problems. A few core principles are underlying this treatment that you should know about. This is the premise by which to approach CBT.

1. Psychological problems are based in part on faulty, unhelpful ways of thinking.
2. Psychological problems are based in part on learned patterns of unhelpful behavior.
3. People suffering from psychological problems can learn better ways of coping with them, thereby relieving their symptoms and becoming more effective in their lives.

As you can tell, CBT treatment is very active and hands-on with your thinking patterns. It is goal-oriented and requires collaboration between you and your therapist with the ultimate goal of becoming your own coach and therapist once you've mastered how to get a handle on your thoughts, feelings, and behavior.

How CBT can help:

- It can help you identify the root problems causing your anxiety with clarity.
- You'll develop an awareness of your automatic thoughts.
- It will help you become aware of and challenge the underlying assumptions running your life that may be wrong.
- You'll be able to distinguish between facts and irrational thoughts.
- You will understand how past experiences can affect present feelings and beliefs.
- It will enable you to stop fearing the worst.
- You will start to see the situations in your daily life from a different perspective.
- It will give you the ability to understand other people's actions and motivations.
- You'll develop a more positive way of thinking and seeing situations.
- It will help you face your fears instead of avoiding them.
- You'll become more aware of your mood and state of mind.
- It helps you establish attainable goals.

- You will learn strategies for managing challenging moments or triggers as they arise.

The tools most used in CBT include role-playing activities, homework assignments, keeping a cognitive-behavioral diary, practicing the skills learned to promote positive behavioral change and growth, and regular one-to-one or group discussion sessions (usually it's a combination of these).

While most traditional therapy involves indefinite visits and time spent on the couch passively digging up your past, Cognitive Behavioral Therapy is timed and focuses on present thoughts and beliefs. As you go through CBT and learn to change your perception and how you see things in your life, your relationship with anxiety, and learn more about who you really are, the outcome will be a shift for the better.

THE IMPACT CBT CAN HAVE ON YOUR LIFE:

With cognitive behavior therapy, you stand to learn that while you cannot control every aspect of the world or change the past, you can, in fact, take control of how you interpret and deal with things in your environment. CBT will help you learn strategies that'll empower and aid you now and in the future, including identifying negative thoughts, goal setting, problem-solving, self-monitoring, and so much more. Let's briefly look at each of the key strategies and how they can help.

Self-monitoring:

One of the first things you'll have to do in CBT is to start monitoring yourself. That means tracking your behavior, symptoms, and experiences over time and then sharing them with your therapist. Some people like to call it diary work. Doing this will help both you and the therapist clarify what's needed so you can be on the best treatment possible. It also allows you to make adjustments where necessary. An example of this would be to keep track of the environment, any triggers, emotions, and what you're doing when a panic attack occurs.

Setting goals:

Goal setting is going to be an essential step in your recovery. If you don't set the right goal and have a target to move toward, how can you possibly know if your life is getting better? So, in CBT, your therapist can help you with goal-setting skills by teaching you how to identify the right goals for you and create short and long-term milestones. A method I like to use and recommend you take up is setting S.M.A.R.T goals. These are Specific. Measurable. Attainable. Relevant. Time-based goals. Once you have it, focus on the process and enjoy the journey till the desired outcome is achieved.

Identifying negative thoughts:

In cognitive-behavioral therapy, you will learn the importance of recognizing dominant thoughts and emotions that rule your life. As you gain this awareness, you'll start to see how thoughts, feelings, and situations can contribute to maladaptive behaviors. This process isn't necessarily easy. In fact, many people struggle with this much introspection which is why it's a good idea to do it with a health professional, so you don't fall off track or dig yourself into an inescapable hole. When done correctly, this will lead to self-discovery and insights that will liberate you from your anxiety.

Problem-solving:

Problem-solving in CBT typically involves five steps. The first is identifying the problem. The second is generating a list of possible solutions. The third is evaluating the strengths and weaknesses of each possible solution. The fourth step involves choosing a solution to implement. The fifth step is implementing the solution and sticking with it until the desired outcome is achieved.

PRACTICE MINDFULNESS WITH DIALECTICAL BEHAVIOR THERAPY (DBT)

Dialectical Behavioral Therapy is another option for helping you heal anxiety forever. It has evolved from cognitive behavioral therapy. Therefore, many of the core principles apply here. Its main goal is to teach you how to live-in-the-moment and develop healthy ways to cope with stress, regulate your emotions and improve your relationship. It focuses on mindfulness or living in the present, regulating emotions, tolerating distress, and effectively managing relationships with others.

DBT incorporates a philosophical process called dialectics. Dialectics is a Greek philosophical concept that states everything is composed of opposites and that change occurs when there is a "dialogue" between opposing forces. There are three basic assumptions to consider here:

1. All things are interconnected.
2. Change is constant and inevitable.
3. Opposites can be integrated to form a closer approximation of the truth.

So, with DBT, you and the therapist would work together to resolve the contradiction between self-acceptance and change to bring about the desired positive outcome. You would also use a technique known as validation which means your therapist will validate that your actions "make sense" within the context of your personal experiences without necessarily agreeing with that approach of solving the existing problem.

THE IMPACT DBT CAN HAVE ON YOUR LIFE:

Suppose you suffer from multiple forms of anxiety and other self-destructive behavior. In that case, this might be the right therapy for you. A unique aspect of DBT that makes it so effective is that it helps you practice self-acceptance. You learn to deal with distress and difficulties in a compassionate way instead of trying to fight or hide them. With DBT, you will learn mindfulness skills, distress tolerance, interpersonal effectiveness, and emotional regulation. Let's touch on these core strategies so you can see how they can be applied.

Core Mindfulness:

Mindfulness helps you focus on being present. It's about living in the moment and paying attention to what is happening inside you, i.e., your thoughts, feelings, sensations, and impulses. You also learn to use your senses to tune into what's happening around you. Mindfulness skills help you slow down as you learn to use healthy coping strategies amid emotional pain. It can also be used to keep you calm and avoid engaging in automatic negative thought patterns and impulsive behavior.

Distress Tolerance:

This is a powerful aspect of DBT because you learn to accept yourself and the current unpleasant situation instead of resisting it, which usually makes things worse. You will discover four techniques for handling any crisis. Distraction, improving the moment, self-soothing, and thinking of the pros and cons of not tolerating distress.

Emotional regulation:

Regulating your emotions is one of the best tools you can have as you move forward in life. You'll learn how to identify, name, and change your feelings whenever the need arises. For example, suppose you're going about your day shopping in the supermarket, and an incident occurs with the cashier that throws you off your game. In that case, you can be able to recognize what that emotion is (e.g., anger) and cope with it immediately, reducing your emotional vulnerability. That alone can help you deactivate many of the triggers that await you as you go through life and helps you have more positive emotional experiences because you can finally control what you choose to feel at any given moment regardless of external conditions.

Interpersonal Effectiveness:

Here you will learn how to nurture healthy relationships. If you struggle with being assertive and saying no when it needs to be said, this is where you develop that level of confidence to be yourself. You will learn how to become a better listener, how to communicate more effectively, and how to deal with toxic or challenging people.

ACT WITH ACCEPTANCE COMMITMENT THERAPY (ACT)

Acceptance Commitment Therapy is often referred to as the "third wave" of psychotherapy. In this context, the first wave would be the classical conditioning and operant learning-based behavioral approaches that were developed in the 1950s. Therefore, the second wave would be the more information processing type of therapy where cognitive processes and behavioral learning principles take center stage. Naturally, the third wave would be ACT. With this "third wave" of psychotherapy (which has become extremely popular for treating general anxiety disorders), the emphasis is on mindfulness, practicing empathy, compassion, and self-acceptance.

As the name implies, this form of therapy focuses on acceptance. ACT (Acceptance Commitment Therapy) suggests that increasing acceptance of your circumstance instead of resisting it can lead to increased psychological flexibility. Rather than avoid specific thoughts, emotions, or experiences, acceptance can better help you cope with things more effectively. So, using this form of treatment, you will gain insight into patterns of thinking and avoidance that have been worsening your anxiety disorder. You will also see the presence and absence of actions that fall in line with your personal values.

What stands out for me with ACT is that, unlike CBT or DBT, this form of treatment doesn't focus on reducing the frequency of unpleasant internal disturbance (e.g., cognitive distortion/irrational thoughts). Instead, it's about decreasing your need to control or eradicate these experiences while simultaneously increasing involvement in meaningful life activities, i.e., the things that are consistent with your personal values.

THE IMPACT ACT CAN HAVE IN YOUR LIFE:

There are six core principles of acceptance and commitment therapy: cognitive defusion, acceptance, observing self, contact with the present moment, values, and committed action. Let's touch on each of these.

Cognitive defusion:

Cognitive defusion is learning to detach yourself from sensations, thoughts, memories, urges, images, feelings, and thoughts that harm you. ACT teaches you how to stop fighting against and resist these unpleasant inner experiences and instead reduce their influence on you. Working with a therapist, he or she will help you see how struggling against negative thoughts is like trying to climb out of quicksand. The harder you try, the worse you make your situation. Most of the time, therapists will use metaphors that apply to your situation and then show you how to use acceptance and commitment to make things better. One of the techniques you'll be taught is how to reframe some of the thoughts that show up. For example, suppose you suffer from social anxiety disorder and usually try to cope using unhealthy strategies like drinking alcohol. In that case, you'll come to see how trying to control your anxiety is part of the problem instead of the solution.

Your therapists may also ask you to say what you're thinking and feeling. If you usually have thoughts like "Everyone thinks I'm boring," then your therapist will ask you to reframe that to "I'm having the thought that everyone thinks I am boring "... You can add the words "I have the thought..." at the beginning of every thought that isn't constructive. This gives you some detachment and reduces the impact your thoughts have so you can realize you are not your thoughts.

As you come to realize that you are neither your thoughts nor the mind, you can more naturally imagine that your feelings, thoughts, and images are just soldiers in a parade passing by but having little impact on you.

The observing self:

This is going to be a powerful tool that your therapist will teach you to utilize. It involves learning to notice that you can observe your thoughts, emotions, and environment. You will learn to see that you are in control of your thoughts and feelings. They are not dangerous, threatening, or more powerful than you. Can you imagine how liberating it will be to detach yourself from intrusive thoughts or painful emotional experiences when they attack? Nothing will ever have a strong grip on you once you take back your power and become the observer.

Acceptance:

Learning to accept unwanted experiences and things that you cannot control will significantly reduce your anxiety. It's common to find your therapist using phrases like "clean discomfort" and "dirty discomfort." Clean discomfort refers to normal feelings of anxiety when the situation calls for it, such as feeling anxious in social and performance situations. Dirty discomfort refers to what happens when anxiety is triggered by your own hyperactivity, such as becoming anxious because your anxiety is increasing. A typical exercise that many people go through involves a guided visualization where the therapist asks you to imagine that you have a switch in the back of your brain. When that switch is "ON," you will struggle and fight against any unpleasant experience, making things worse. You may become angry, sad, and anxious about the increasing anxiety. These emotions are known as secondary emotions, and they usually set up a vicious cycle. So, your therapist will ask you to switch "OFF" that button and notice what happens. As you become present and pay attention, you'll see these secondary emotions will dissipate.

Values:

Do you know who you really are and what you stand for? What is important to you in life? What has meaning in your life? Is it family? Faith? Can you identify it? Getting to know your values can help you set the right health goals and ensure you follow a treatment that ensures permanent results.

Working with an ACT therapist, you will uncover your values and identify whether you're living in integrity with those values and what adjustments need to be made. That is extremely valuable for treating anxiety because a lot of research points to low self-esteem and other value-based factors as one of the many causes that could lead to anxiety disorders.

Committed action:

As you go through the treatment, you will be asked to commit yourself to action that is in line with your values. This might cause uneasiness at first, especially if you have drifted too far from your natural state. But you must commit and implement.

One of the powerful strategies you will learn during ACT treatment is how to practice non-judgmental awareness. You'll learn to understand your emotions at a whole new level and to observe without judging yourself harshly.

Additionally, you'll also be involved in a lot of mindfulness exercises. Through mindfulness practices that run deeper than what you learn in DBT, you'll develop the tools and skills needed to maintain calm and to practice non-resistance whenever you're faced with a challenging situation or irrational thoughts.

A CHANGE IN LIFESTYLE GOES A LONG WAY

Recovering and healing from major anxiety will require a change in your current lifestyle and the habits that aren't serving you. This could mean getting back into the habit of doing things that you used to but lost interest in, or it could be learning something entirely new.

I recently watched famous actress Halley Berry talk about the training she had to undergo for six months to prepare for her role, starring alongside Keanu Reeves in John Wick 3. She said it was tough to condense into six months what would typically take regular people three years to learn, but there was no quitting and no complaining. Only showing up and getting the work done.

You don't need to be so insane about it and try to do the impossible, but in a way, you will need that same persistent mindset for a period of time (at least six months) where your only focus is sticking to the habits you know will help you transform your life. For example, if you used to exercise but gave up on it when your anxiety or depression became too intense, restarting that habit will need a lot of self-motivation. And just like Halley Berry, you need to sell yourself into this idea of training so much that you refuse to accept any thoughts of quitting, giving up, or complaining. You will need to show up for yourself each day to get the work done, no matter how uncomfortable it feels. You also need to keep trying new things, including learning new hobbies that help you express your creativity, challenge your brainpower, and so on. Now, I realize that at times even getting out of bed in the morning feels like a herculean task. And I know some days you might have dips of depression or panic attacks that completely disrupt your stamina, but I still want you to do your best even on your worst days. Why?

Because the only way to transform your life is to show yourself that you can control how you feel and behave. Your lifestyle choices can either help make things better or worse. Here are some lifestyle shifts that are scientifically proven to work in reducing or completely eliminating anxiety disorders.

Good quality sleep: Most of us think we get enough rest, but our society, in general, is sleep-deprived, so it's no surprise that we need to put more effort into getting better quality sleep. If you go to bed and spend an hour browsing social media or chatting on WhatsApp, then try to fall asleep, your sleep quality will likely be compromised. Anytime you are stressed and anxious, your body will naturally require more rest and relaxation. Sleep is a great way to get the body to rest, but you need to ensure the environment fosters good quality rest. Unfortunately, as you may have experienced already, anxiety makes it hard for us to find that state of good quality rest and relaxation. So even if I go to bed early (without any gadgets to distract me), but I can't fall asleep because I am anxious for half the night; I'm still not going to be well-rested the next morning. And since many people suffering from anxiety tend to have insomnia, telling someone to simply go to bed early won't cut it. So how can you start changing your sleep habits?

Realize that it doesn't help to stay up late binge-watching Netflix or Amazon Prime. But at the same time, you shouldn't force yourself to go to bed too early. Learn to listen to your body. Start to practice what experts call sleep hygiene. That means you need to create a good and relaxing bedtime routine and then stick to it. You should also make your bedroom as relaxing and sleep-friendly as possible. Some little changes you could start with today include putting an end to anything that stimulates your brain at least an hour before your bedtime—no television, computers, coffee, cigarettes, or anything that stimulates wakefulness. If you love drinking something after dinner, switch the coffee to herbal tea.

Exercising: Regular exercise is one of the best things you can do to reduce anxiety symptoms and promote healing. Studies conducted show that physical movement and breaking a sweat can boost your mood, improve your sleep quality, reduce tension in your body, and lower stress levels. The more you exercise, the more energy your body generates, which will benefit you in so many ways, including increasing your ability to concentrate. There are many forms of exercise depending on your preference, but I highly recommend taking some Yoga classes a few times a week. The combination of mindfulness breathing and physically moving your body has been linked to reducing anxiety symptoms. I recommend making a commitment to spend just twenty minutes daily on some form of exercise that you enjoy even a little bit. That is ample time to activate your endorphins which is the body's natural mood booster.

Good nutrition: Although there's no specific type of food you can eat to eliminate anxiety, we do know that having a healthy, well-balanced diet can help you during the recovery process. Stimulants containing caffeine and other substances that have a tendency of sending your body into hyperactivity will need to be avoided or eliminated.

Maintain a healthy eating routine and snack at regular intervals to help your body adjust and cope with the treatment and healing process. Also, consider reducing the amount of processed and junk food that you consume. Raw, simple foods will serve your body and boost your energy far more than junk foods. A diet rich in whole grains, vegetables, and fruits is a healthier option that I recommend focusing on, so here is a list of foods that have been shown to reduce anxiety.

- Foods rich in zinc such as cashews, beef, egg yolks, and oysters have been linked to lowered anxiety levels.
- Magnesium-rich foods such as leafy greens like Swiss chard and Spinach or nuts, seeds, legumes, and whole grains should be part of your daily intake.
- Foods rich in B vitamins such as avocado and almonds have also been associated with lowered anxiety levels.
- A study completed on medical students in 2011 showed that omega-3s may help reduce anxiety. Consider adding fatty fish like wild Alaskan salmon to your meal planning.

Since anxiety is thought to be correlated with a lowered antioxidant state, consider adding beans, berries, and vegetables (beets, broccoli, kale, artichokes, and asparagus) to your diet, as well as spices like turmeric and ginger, which contain antioxidant properties.

Proper hydration: Multiple studies show a correlation between dehydration and anxiety. In one 2018 survey of over 3,000 adults, those who drank more water had a lower risk of anxiety and depression than those who drank less water (source: Healthline.com). We know through firsthand experience that lack of proper hydration messes with brain functionality. The brain, which is composed mainly of water, requires a lot of it to perform optimally. So, people who drink lots of water usually feel calmer and happier. There's a lot of increased tension, a drop in focus, and mood when one doesn't hydrate enough, making anxiety levels worsen. But how do you know you're dehydrated, and how much water should you take anyway? The first signs of dehydration are thirst, a dry mouth, dark yellow urine, constipation, skin changes, including dryness, redness, or loss of turgor. You might also experience sleepiness, fatigue, confusion, headache, nausea, or even high blood pressure.

The Academy of Nutrition and Dietetics suggests that women should drink around 9 cups of water every day while men to consume around 12.5 cups. Of course, this should not be a fixed number because each body is different. Start with a fixed number and get to learn what your body thrives in. Depending on your activity levels, age, and how much water you usually take through foods like fruit and vegetables, your daily water intake may vary.

If you find water drinking to be a task too great for you, consider setting the alarm on your phone each hour to get in a cup. It's a great way to establish this as a permanent habit.

II

PRACTICAL TECHNIQUES
AND YOUR PERSONAL GUIDE
ON OVERCOMING YOUR
ANXIETY AND PANIC
ATTACKS

5

CREATE A MORNING ROUTINE TO START REDUCING ANXIETY RIGHT AT THE BEGINNING OF YOUR DAY

I t's time to get into strategies that will help you get your life back. You now have a working understanding of what happens when anxiety or panic kicks in and the leading causes. With that foundation in place, we can start taking baby steps in the right direction. This section of the book will help establish a couple of necessary pillars: your body, mind, and environment.

It should be evident by now that your body and mind are interconnected. What you feel and say to yourself impacts your body positively or negatively. The environment you spend the most time in also influences your body and mind. Therefore, the path to recovery involves being more proactive in these three aspects. But let's break them down further into bite-sized changes you can make, starting with how you approach your day.

THE IMPORTANCE OF STARTING THE DAY WITH A MORNING ROUTINE

How you start the morning determines the rest of the day. We all know how tough it can be to get the day started right, so one of the most significant shifts you can implement immediately is to create a morning routine designed to promote harmony, relaxation, and ease. Studies show that a change in morning routine for a person struggling with anxiety reduces the chances of an episode both in the morning and later in the day. It also helps increase awareness of the triggers that usually lead to an anxiety attack.

A good morning routine will bring about a sense of harmony, relaxation, and stability to your body and mind. It will give you the confidence you need to feel more in control of your emotions and, ultimately, your thoughts. Although I'm not a believer in the cookie-cutter approach or a one-size-fits-all strategy for morning routines, I want to make it as easy for you to get going as I can. That means sharing a blueprint or as many ideas as possible so you can custom make your own or imitate precisely what I share. Listen, I know it can be hard to try anything new when battling major anxiety issues, but you don't even have to think about it with what I'm sharing. Read the instructions and apply. Try whichever one feels more comfortable and discard those that don't feel right for you.

Wake up earlier

A great morning routine that sets you up for success cannot be rushed. It will take at least 60 minutes, sometimes longer. But the first shift you need to make is adjusting your bedtime so you can wake up at least 30 minutes earlier for the next week or two. In time, you'll find it easier to wake up at your perfect time, where the morning routine flows without the need to rush or skip essential things.

Morning Gratitude

When you become consciously aware that a brand new day has started for you, I encourage you to think of three things you feel grateful for. Do this even before you open your eyes. Mentally think of these three things or speak them out loud if convenient. The act of thanksgiving as the first thing you do in the morning will lift your spirits and lighten your mood. It will help you get out of bed on the right foot and keep negativity at bay.

Hydrate

We addressed the importance of drinking plenty of water. Your brain needs a lot of water to function at optimal levels, and when you sleep, you lose a lot of water naturally. So, we all wake up a little dehydrated. Add a mental disorder to that dehydration, and it's easy to see why getting up feels daunting. Yet that's what you need to do. By drinking a glass of water immediately after waking up, you hydrate the body and brain and get your juices flowing in all the right ways. What I developed over the years is the habit of drinking water with some freshly squeezed lemon first thing in the morning. Lemon water has many added benefits, but even a plain glass of water will serve just as good. The most important thing to remember is to hydrate with something natural—no coffee or even tea at this point.

Wash Up

Most people think this is obvious, but even a shower can feel like a giant task when in the midst of battling anxiety. Some might even procrastinate and skip showers, so I need you to see this as part of your morning routine. Brush teeth, floss and scrape your tongue. Take a nice hot or cold shower. In short, get yourself nice and clean. Practicing this kind of self-care and body hygiene sends a positive message to your brain and increases those feel-good hormones.

Move Your Body

I like to get my workout done before jumping into my day because I am less likely to procrastinate if I do it early in the morning. Suppose you prefer to exercise in the afternoon or later in the day. In that case, I still encourage you to do some form of body movement within the first hour. It can be a five to ten-minute stretch or yoga flow. You can also do some skipping, jumping jacks, dancing, squats, pushups, or anything that gets your blood pumping.

Journaling

Daily thought recording and capturing your emotions are going to be an essential part of your recovery. Journaling in the morning is one way you can track your recovery and take control of your day. It's a great habit to develop, especially if you want to train your mind to think thoughts that put you in a calm and comfortable state for the day ahead.

Meditate

We will be discussing mindfulness practices and mediation at length in an upcoming chapter. Still, I wanted to include it here because it is part of my morning routine. I have found meditation to be the best way for me to take command of my day. I get to slow down my body and bring myself back to a state of calm and ease. It's literally the best feeling in the world. I've been practicing this for years, so don't worry if, in the beginning, you spend all your time wandering away from one thought to another. Once you get the hang of it, I think it will play a significant role in your healing. The amount of time you spend in meditation should depend on your personality and temperament. As a beginner, even 1 minute of daily meditation is better than nothing. You could eventually build up to five minutes daily. An ideal time to strive for would be 15 minutes.

Dress to Impress Yourself

Spending all day in your pajamas or unflattering clothes, whether you work from home or not, can induce that feeling of lethargy. Even if you don't work at a formal office whereby a suit and tie are required, I want you to always dress up. Put on clothes that make you feel good. Brush your hair, and if you like, put on a little make-up (if that's your thing). Anything that makes you feel good will activate the right hormones and help you stay in the right state for most of the day. One thing to note here is that you should wear something comfortable that makes you feel great, not something that impresses others!

Read

Reading something spiritually uplifting or inspiring is one of the best-kept secrets for transforming your life and aiding your recovery. Are you a person of strong faith? Invest ten minutes each morning reading a devotional or the Bible. Do you find certain teachers, business moguls, or topics inspiring? Invest in those books and read with some tea in hand for a few minutes. Allow yourself to feed your mind with food that nourishes and promotes productivity.

These are simple things you can do. The order in which I stated them shouldn't be taken into consideration. What matters is that you integrate them into your life appropriately. Perhaps you just looked at my list and wondered how you can possibly do all these things given your current demanding schedule. In that case, here's a quick practice that can still work, and it only takes a few minutes.

THE BEST 10-MINUTE DAILY PRACTICE TO RAPIDLY REDUCE YOUR ANXIETY AT THE START OF EVERY DAY!

Suppose you seriously cannot add more than ten minutes to your morning, but you want something that will help you reduce anxiety. In that case, my best recommendation is to commit to ten-minute meditation practice. One that has been specifically designed to impact you powerfully.

The unique thing about meditating as a quick morning routine to alleviate anxiety is that you get the added bonus of improving other areas making it a holistic approach to your recovery. Both science and spirituality show that meditation will help you become more stable and focused. You will develop the ability to remain more present throughout the day and increase your sense of compassion, kindness, patience, and joy. Besides that, medication will improve your overall physical health, increase productivity, and lower stress levels. Although you could meditate anytime during the day or before going to sleep, the following guided meditation is best practiced first thing in the morning.

The scripted meditation below walks you through the step-by-step practice for calming your mind, including stabilizing your breath, letting go of unpleasant thoughts, and watching your posture.

Begin by finding a quiet and comfortable spot in your home. Settle yourself into a meditation posture. You can sit cross-legged on an elevated cushion or upright and comfortable in your favorite chair with your feet flat on the floor and your palms facing upwards and resting on your lap. Gently touch the tips of your thumb and index finger on each hand. Straighten your spine and tilt your head toward the floor to find a focus point. Make sure your shoulders and neck are relaxed. Let go of any tension in your face, neck, shoulders, and throughout your body. Half close your eyes and slightly open your mouth.

Think for a moment the main reason for entering into this mediation. Perhaps you want to address some stress or anxiety or sleeplessness or worry. Notice for a moment that you desire to take away these problems. Feel compassion for yourself rising within you as you connect with that desire of returning your mind to its natural state of peace and happiness.

You may also want to meditate so you can bring out more of your best human features. The qualities of kindness, compassion, generosity, patience, and living a life not just to benefit yourself but also help everyone you encounter. Even if it is done through the simple act of smiling at a stranger. Bring that clarity of intention as you enter deeper into this meditation.

Now, bring your attention to your breath. Focus on the breath coming in and out of your nostrils. Notice how cool it is as it comes in and how warm it feels as it goes out. Move your attention to your abdomen. Notice how it rises and falls as you deeply inhale and exhale. If thoughts, bodily sensations, plans, flashbacks, or anything else grabs your attention and you find yourself distracted from focusing on your breathing, that's okay. As soon as you catch yourself, just come back to observing your breathing. Allow these thoughts and sensations to drift by you. And do not feel bad or judge the experience. Mind-wandering is perfectly normal as you learn to meditate. The more you focus on your breathing, the easier it will be for the thoughts and sensations to disappear naturally, just like clouds passing through the sky. Keep focusing on your breathing for a few minutes in silence.

Now, steer your awareness from your breath to your mind. There's still no need to push away your thoughts, and you also don't need to draw them in for examination. But try and notice that there's a part of your mind that's detached from the perceptions coming from your senses. Your eyes, ears, nose, taste, and touch feed you information, but there's more to you than that. There's also a part of your mind that can simply watch and embrace or release thoughts. Notice that this part of your mind isn't the perceptions or the thoughts themselves. Allow this awareness to permeate and fill your attention. Connect with that aspect of yourself naturally... without force, without the need to make anything happen. There's no right or wrong.

As you come closer to experiencing the fullness of your awareness, focus on the space between the thoughts. In the same way, there are gaps between musical notes, so too there exists gaps between thoughts when no thought is present. And you can experience your mind's conscious nature itself. See if you can bring your focus into these gaps and examine what your mind is without them. If you can, gradually expand the gaps between your thoughts so that the thoughts become fewer and fewer, and the intervals of pure awareness get bigger.

Now we can come out of the mediation. Allow your senses to arise again. Notice your senses being reactivated. Feeling sight, taste, smell, touch, and sound activating. Notice any

difference in how you feel. Are you feeling closer to the
present moment? Are you feeling calmer? Are you more at
ease and at peace? Feel that connection to that deeper part
of yourself, beneath the thoughts and perceptions to pure
awareness. In the same way that physical exercise gradually
makes the body healthier, you've just exercised your mind
in a way that gradually makes it calmer and happier.

Feel good now and be proud of yourself because you just invested ten minutes in a practice that will help you cultivate your best human qualities and gradually move toward your best self who is kinder, calmer, more compassionate, and able to forge deep, meaningful connections with others.

MORE PRACTICES THAT YOU CAN ADD TO YOUR MORNING ROUTINE

#1: Avoid checking your phone first thing in the morning:

Most people open their eyes and reach for their phone even before getting out of bed. They get bombarded with messages, emails, and the temptation to scroll through social media to catch what they missed while sleeping. For people dealing with anxiety, this is a recipe for disaster.

If you charge your phone by your bed or use it as an alarm clock, you'll likely end up consumed by the alerts and news that await you. Before you know it, you're sucked in, and a quick scroll turns into the 20 minutes you had for self-care. I recommend charging your phone as far away from your bed as possible. Make sure it is not within reach. If you can leave all your gadgets outside your bedroom area, that's even better. Smartphones have transformed the way we communicate, and that's great. But they have also become a massive source of anxiety for everyone. Adding a new rule to detach from your phone the night before and allowing the first minutes of the day to be a distraction and phone-free time can significantly impact your mood and how calm you feel during your self-care morning routine. This is especially necessary if you have a demanding career or if you usually wake up, check your phone, and already feel anxious for the day ahead.

#2: Do some morning visualization and set clear intentions for your day:

It might seem too simple, but trust me, setting an intention of how you want to feel on this brand new day can help you maintain a calm state. And if you don't want to stretch it by affirming the whole day, then just make an intention for how you want to feel in the morning. Sit for a few minutes, either after breakfast or before leaving the house, and spend a few minutes visualizing how you want your morning or day to go. Set an intentional tone and feel yourself moving through the day in that calm, focused, and empowered state. Consider recalling a memory that evokes the kind of feeling you want to have in this new day. For example, I usually sit for a few minutes before leaving for the office and remember a fond memory of me on the peak of a mountain overlooking the summit. I had gone hiking up a mountain with some friends, and it was an incredible experience. I can vividly recall the details of the scenery, how peaceful and powerful

I felt. The sounds of nature that surrounded me made it seem like I was floating about everything else. I felt so proud and accomplished and unstoppable after making that long and challenging trek to the top. Now I bring that memory to life each morning, and it does wonders to my confidence and sense of empowerment. Now it's your turn. Can you think of a specific memory that brings out similar emotions? Allow yourself to soak in that memory and build that same intention into each new day, even if you're spending the day in an office building.

#3: Add some essential oils to your shower:

A soothing shower in the morning is essential if you want to have a great morning. But I want you to take it a step further and invest in some soothing essential oils that you can add to your shower. It is the perfect antidote to anxiety because essential oils are known to calm down the senses and release tension in the body. It adds that much-needed feeling of self-care in the morning routine. Think of it as a personalized spa experience. Oils like lavender, chamomile, frankincense contain properties that promote a sense of ease, so pick a smell that resonates with you and make this part of your morning shower. You could even have a particular essential oil for the morning shower to get you invigorated and ready to take on the day and then a special one for the evening that enables you to unwind and prepare for a peaceful sleep. While using essential oils in the shower, make sure to practice some deep breathing. Take slow deep breaths and enjoy tuning into your sense of smell. Through this simple practice, you will be activating lots of positive practices all at the same time, including personal hygiene and self-care practices as well as mindfulness practices through deep breathing.

MAKING THOSE MORNING ROUTINES STICK EFFECTIVELY

The hardest part of making your morning routine stick is to figure out what works best for you. It's not merely a question of willpower or discipline. It's also about asking yourself what you genuinely enjoy and what aligns with your current lifestyle. For example, if you have young children, it's rather challenging to carve out an hour in the morning for your self-care and morning ritual. If you have a long commute to work, it's also challenging to do many of the things gurus claim must be done in the morning for optimal performance. So, the first thing I would do is look at your lifestyle, the daily demands that you need to meet, and then ask yourself, "what do I enjoy doing, and how much time can I commit for myself each morning?" So, if you only have 20 minutes for your morning routine, that's perfectly okay. I prefer having 20 minutes daily doing something that makes me feel good instead of waking up at 4 am in the morning and cut my sleep short just to have a full hour of activities I don't particularly enjoy. Especially if I'm doing it because a guru told me it works. See where I'm going with this?

Everything I shared in this chapter may or may not be enjoyable for you. It's upon you to take that initiative, personalize what feels right for you, and then do it consistently. If you only have twenty minutes, mix and match a bit of reading with some light stretches and meditation. If you enjoy the idea of a nice shower with essential oils, then add that as well.

To make your routine stick, you will need to experiment with a few suggestions until you figure out the best fit for you.

A good starting place might be taking notice of your biggest stressors and problems that trigger your anxiety, then consider morning activities that might help alleviate them. If, for example, you get anxious as soon as you think about the day ahead and all the things you have to do, then consider journaling first thing in the morning, write down a simple plan of execution for the day, do some light visualization, and set your intention for the day.

Make it as easy as possible, so you stick with this new morning ritual. The first few weeks of your new routine matter the most because this is when the habit forms. Experts recommend writing down the main activities and sticking them around the house (on the mirror, fridge, laptop) where you can easily see them so they can stay top of mind.

You can also use your alarm as a reminder. For example, if you've committed to a 30 minute virtual workout at 7.30 am, then your alarm should go off at 7.25am, alerting you to be ready in five minutes. After a few days, you'll find your body clock will start getting into the rhythm, and you may not need an alarm. The same goes for drinking water at various points during the day. Use that smartphone for something other than social media and internet surfing!

You should also set clear and specific goals with your morning routine and try to do the same activities at the same time each day. For example, instead of saying I will work out every morning before breakfast, decide what time you will work out, how long the workout will last, and which activity it will be. You can also prepare the night before little reminders and triggers to get you into a particular habit. If you enjoy having some tea before showering and you'd like to use that time to journal, place your diary right next to the teapot the night before. This will enable each activity to serve as a cue for the next one. In time, the habit will form. It will flow naturally as long as you enjoy integrating that activity into your life.

If you are seeing a therapist or have a support group, that's also a great way to receive the encouragement you need to stick with your routine. Let your support team know what you are doing and allow them to become accountability partners checking up on you regularly to make sure you're not cheating your way out of recovery.

EXAMPLES OF GREAT MORNING ROUTINES THAT ARE EASY TO ADAPT:

Kristy's nutritious breakfast combined with mindful eating:

Kristy realized that emphasizing a nutritious breakfast and practicing mindfulness helped create a calm and productive morning. She says that she sits and mindfully eats a nutritious breakfast as part of a calm start to the day. Kristy shares that she feels energized and more stable mentally and physically when she includes healthy fats, protein, and slow-releasing carbs into her breakfast meal choice.

How to make your breakfast nutritious and enjoyable:

Consider smoked salmon on seeded whole grain bread, a good source of vitamin D and Omega-3 fatty acids. You can also opt for eggs with spinach to boost essential amino acids that help your brain produce dopamine and serotonin. If you're a fruit lover, berry chia puddings are a great nutritious option. You could also go for almonds and yogurt with probiotics. Are you a porridge fan? How about having some oats with banana and nut butter, or alternatively, you could go for oatcakes topped with avocado. For a vegan option, consider adding turmeric to your tofu. Regardless of your breakfast choice, make sure you eat mindfully.

Julie's mindful morning self-care routine:

Julie's routine begins with a mindful appreciation routine, a mindful shower, some stretches, and a quick meditation. With the mindful appreciation, Julie spends five minutes upon waking up to reflect on one thing she's happily anticipating. Some days, that one thing is hopping back to bed at the end of the day! So, it's not about something extraordinary. Instead, it's the act of simple gratitude first thing in the morning. You could feel thankful that you have a bed and a home, a healthy body, or even the fact that despite your current challenges, you are still alive.

Energetically, that positive appreciation feeling sets a mood for the rest of the morning. Julie also says she enjoys using her sense of smell to invigorate her. Her morning ritual includes a calming shower gel and a specifically chosen scent that she applies to her body. That scent has the power to transform her mood instantly. By taking a warm shower, practicing mindfulness while in the shower, and then investing a few minutes in oiling her entire body with a pleasurable aroma, Julie can encourage, invigorate and motivate herself into a good feeling state.

Consider experimenting with scents like peppermint, lavender, pine, myrrh, or rose, depending on your personal taste. Think about how you would like to feel all day, and then pick a scent that matches that feeling. For example, if you want to feel calm and relaxed, myrrh or lavender is recommended.

6

THE ALMOST UNKNOWN HEALING POWER OF BREATHWORK AND COLD-WATER THERAPY FOR OBLITERATING YOUR ANXIETY

W e've discussed therapy and the different forms known to effectively deal with anxiety and panic attacks. Getting into treatment and combining that with other lifestyle changes that promote health and wellbeing could be the key to healing your life forever. Unfortunately, therapy comes with a significant drawback. If you don't have health insurance or the finances to foot the bill, it's not a plausible solution. For many people, the thought of paying for a therapist only exacerbates their anxiety because of the costs involved. So, what can you do if you're not in a position to invest in a therapist?

This book has already introduced you to the main psychotherapeutic treatments the therapist would guide you through. Combine that knowledge with what you're about to learn in this chapter, and you should already notice a difference in your condition. And by the way, what I am about to share can be viewed as a form of therapy, except this one is 100% free.

Breathwork and how to use it as your meditation practice:

Ever heard of the term breathwork? It's a general term used to refer to any breathing technique or exercise that emphasizes using your breath to improve your mental, physical and spiritual state. Most practices take about twenty minutes to an hour of sustained rhythmic breathing.

Many therapy forms incorporate breathwork, each with its own unique approach. Some are easy to do at home, while others will require a practitioner to guide you. Breathwork is inspired by Eastern practices like Tai Chi and yoga, which, as you know, really help the body utilize the breath to bring about radical transformation. In breathwork, the main emphasis should be to raise your self-aware-ness. It can take the form of talk therapy, breathing exercises, art, music, and bodywork.

As a form of therapy, breathwork has shown positive results when treating anxiety which is why you're going to learn how to incorpo-rate breathwork into your daily routine. There are many forms of breathwork therapy, most of which are founded on similar principles. The best ones include:

Biodynamic Breathwork

The biodynamic breath and trauma release system integrates six elements: breath, movement, sound, touch, emotion, and meditation. The purpose of this is to release tension, support natural healing, and restructure internal systems. Through this approach, balance is restored to your entire system. Treatment includes exercises like deep, connected breathing, revisiting ingrained memories and sensations. It can also include music or sound therapy, whole body shaking, vocalization, and dance therapy.

Holotropic Breathwork

This form of breathwork is concerned with achieving wholeness of mind, body, and spirit. Evocative music and occasional bodywork are used as you perform specific breathing exercises while lying down. In this particular breathwork, you would also create mandalas related to your breathwork experience immediately after the breathing exercises. That will help you integrate what you learn about yourself during the session.

While there are several other forms, let's discuss some breathwork exercises that you can do immediately.

- *Box breathing.* That involves taking slow, deep breathes to the count of four, holding your breath for another count of four, and then slowly exhaling for a count of four.
- *Continuous circular breathing.* That involves using full deep breaths in and out continuously. You don't need to hold your breath at any point. Instead, you want to create a circular rhythm that symbolizes the circle of breath.
- *Immersion in water.* That involves immersing yourself in water and either breathing deeply above the surface of the water or with the aid of a snorkel.
- *20 connected breaths.* That involves breathing in and out 20 times. Here, you would take four sets of four short breaths

and one deep breath. The breathing should be done through the nose unless you're unable due to specific medical reasons.

WHY PRACTICE DEEP BREATHING OR BREATHWORK?

There are many benefits of practicing this form of therapy. Studies show that even a few deep breaths can lower blood pressure and cortisol levels and increase parasympathetic tone. Take your deep breathing to the next level by incorporating breathwork. You get a whole new level of benefits, including mood elevation, decreased stress and anxiety, increased self-awareness, and an overall feeling of joy and happiness.

It's important to note here that while I recommend doing this with a combination of meditation, it shouldn't substitute your morning routine meditation because they are, in essence, different practices with different objectives. So, when you practice your deep breathing exercise as you meditate, make it intentionally geared toward the breathwork technique and not as a way of stilling the mind, as is usually the case with regular meditation.

USING COLD WATER DURING BATH TIME

Besides breathwork, there's another little-known (and also free) therapy known as hydrotherapy. It is a simple remedy that you can do immediately and receive great benefits. Hydrotherapy involves using cold water on your body to help it heal and feel better.

There was a time when we spent a lot of time outdoors. We were continually in contact with nature and directly influenced by changing climate and weather patterns. Although nowadays we barely leave the house save for going to work in an enclosed office or to run grocery errands and such, we can still benefit from some of the insights gained by the experts who found healing properties in natural remedy. One such natural treatment is the use of water. Applying different temperatures to our skin can change our physiology and mood. Did you know that?

Taking a cold swim or doing a "plunge" in a spa with such facilities has shown that the body responds positively. Sure, it's shocking at first, but the cold causes blood circulation to improve in a matter of minutes. The cold shocks the blood vessels, causing vasoconstriction, making the blood move from the surface of your body to the core as a means to conserve heat. This movement brings nutrition and oxygen to the area where circulation is low. It also helps gently detoxify the area. When combined with warm water, the blood vessels vasodilate, bringing blood back to the surface, creating a holistic experience for your entire body. Plenty of medical research has supported the combination of hot and cold baths showing a decrease in stress hormones like cortisol. Evidence also indicates that water bathing helps the balance of the feel-good neurotransmitter serotonin.

Since we know anxiety may cause an increase in blood pressure and inflammation, it's easy to see how a cold shower can help calm your entire nervous system down and promote the release of endorphins in your brain.

When doing this form of therapy at home, I recommend starting with a few minutes at a time, especially if you've never taken cold baths. Consider creating a few rounds of hot and cold and then finishing up the shower with lukewarm water.

DO THEY REALLY WORK?

Breathwork and hydrotherapy have been successful at treating anxiety, but again, it all depends on your particular situation.

A French study suggests patients with anxiety can benefit from the mechanisms of hydrotherapy. Balneotherapy (using water baths for healing) was compared to paroxetine (Paxil), a leading SSRI medication. 237 patients with GAD (generalized anxiety disorder) were assigned randomly to balneotherapy and 120 to the medication. The balneotherapy consisted of weekly medical visits and daily bath treatments using natural mineral water for twenty-one days. How? The patients were immersed in a bubble bath (37 degrees Celsius for ten minutes) then a shower with a firm massage-like pressure targeting the abdomen area along the spine, neck, and arm region for 3 minutes. Finally, the legs, neck and scapular, and spine area would be massaged underwater for another ten minutes. At the end of the duration, both groups showed improvement with a clear superior result for the group that did the water therapy. Remission and sustained response rates were also significantly higher for the hydrotherapy group than the drug group (Dubois et al., 2010).

Regular cold showers can boost your immune system, increase your feel-good hormones and invigorate your brain. That creates the calm state necessary to take back control of your day when anxiety takes over. Breathwork, especially when combined with meditation, is powerful. If done consistently, it will not only increase your awareness, but you will also feel more stable and capable of maintaining an anxiety-free state.

How cold showers and breathwork made an ordinary man seem superhuman:

The famous daredevil and Guinness World Record holder Wim Hof (famously known as the Iceman) has devised a method known as the Wim Hof method (wimhofmethod.com) that combines breathwork and cold showers. He believes anyone can use this method to bring about significant benefits to your entire body. The idea behind it is to combine cold water therapy, breathing, and commitment. Hof believes he has been able to achieve his crazy feats of survival (climbing Kilimanjaro wearing only shorts and shoes, running a half marathon above the Arctic Circle barefoot, and being submerged in an ice bath for 1hr 52 minutes 42 seconds) thanks to his combination of meditation, breathing exercises and exposure to cold as a means of controlling the body's autonomous response systems. By leveraging these simple techniques, you could beat the stress and anxiety that ails you and accelerate your recovery. All you have to do is learn simple breathing techniques (the ones mentioned in this chapter), train yourself to handle some cold water or ice baths and commit to doing it. If you're skeptical about this, give it a try for seven days only. The worst that can happen is that nothing changes. The upside, however, is that you find a simple way to transform your life forever without adding on the cost of buying pricey health supplements or hiring an expensive therapist.

7

WHY YOUR DIET & LIFESTYLE PLAYS A CRITICAL ROLE IN YOUR JOURNEY OF OVERCOMING YOUR ANXIETY DISORDER

Before science became as advanced as we know it today, diet and lifestyle weren't considered necessary in the context of health. I mean, do you know there was a time when cigarette smoking was advertised on television as something good? I know. It's horrifying, but before the 1950s, there wasn't good evidence showing that cigarette smoking was bad for you. So, it wouldn't be uncommon to find ads with doctors endorsing it to the public. Much of this was because our understanding of the human body was minimal.

Today, however, we've made some headway and learned that cigarettes lead to lung cancer, and caffeine doesn't make you smarter! Okay, why am I sharing all this with you? Because it's crucial to develop a proper understanding of how your body works and the impact of your lifestyle choices on your health. In your case, the knowledge you need to get is the connection between your psychological and biological processes. Or stated simply, how your physical body affects your emotional and mental state.

Many people don't realize that there's a link between the physical state and the mental state. It would be impossible to attain permanent healing if we skip over this part, so pay close attention as we uncover the real reason behind the changes I have been recommending with your nutrition and lifestyle.

MIND SHIFT: THINKING OF YOUR PHYSICAL AND MENTAL HEALTH AS ONE

When we realize that we are suffering from a mental disorder, the first and most recommended solution is typically medication, therapy, or some quick fix instead of emphasizing understanding the mind-body connection. That's why I want to invite you to make this shift for yourself, as it is the only way to permanently eradicate the suffering you've had to endure to this point.

What is the connection? The mind - a manifest functioning of the brain - and the other body systems interact in ways critical for health, illness, and wellbeing (Ray, 2004, p.29). Our bodies are intelligent and alive. So whatever signals and messages the brain sends out, the body will respond accordingly. Depending on the dominant thoughts that we allow to set up camp in our minds, corresponding signals that alter our brains will be released to the rest of the body, which will change our biology. That will, in turn, send corresponding feedback to validate the initial message. In no time, you have a feedback loop that solidifies as your normal state. So, if you're stuck in anxious or intrusive thoughts, your brain will release the appropriate hormones and fire neurons that alert the rest of the body that something is wrong.

Blood pressure and heart rate will rise. The body will go into that fight or flight mode, and your physical state will reflect that you experienced anxiety. As the body continues to remain in this distressed state, more corresponding emotions and thoughts will fill your mind. That will elevate your anxiety levels and cause you to feel sick to your stomach. This vicious cycle becomes almost impossible to break, especially if sustained for prolonged periods. The food you consume will also help to exacerbate your state and continue to reinforce your anxiety. Poor mental health leads to poor physical health just as much as poor physical fitness leads to poor mental health. Sometimes it is a chicken and egg situation whereby it's impossible to state which came first. If you suffered from a severe chronic illness as a child or chronic pain due to an accident, that might have activated the disorder. Due to continued poor diet and self-neglect, the disorder grew into a life of its own. It took up residence in your mind and continued to cause damage long after that particular physical condition healed.

As you can see, the starting point might be hard to pinpoint, so don't let that become a priority. What matters is that you are here now and ready to reclaim both your mental and physical health. How do you do this?

A good starting point is with your nutrition. Most people assume getting fit is about working out for hours each day. The truth is, you can get fit and significantly improve your physical health by adjusting your diet first. Then as the diet helps the biology shift, the physiology and psychology will shift too.

A HEALTHY GUT CAN HELP YOU HAVE A HEALTHY MIND

The diet you choose over the next few months will hinder or accelerate your healing. I want you to start viewing your food as medicine and fuel for your body. In Traditional Chinese Medicine, Ayurvedic Medicine, and Native American culture, food has always been an essential aspect of treating illness and maintaining health. An increasing number of studies provide evidence for the curative and preventive properties of certain foods. For example, Green tea is a good source of antioxidants, ginger may be an effective treatment for nausea, and garlic is often used for various things, including to lower cholesterol.

Research from Harvard says food choices can make the difference between feeling worse and feeling more stable. Do you know which foods are actually pro healing? Here are six things you need to drop and five that you need to incorporate into your diet starting now.

#1. Alcohol:

Alcohol is a depressant. More specifically, it depresses the working order of your nervous system, making it challenging to think, reason, understand things or even control your motor function. Oh, and did I mention, your central nervous system processes emotions. So, what happens when you have one too many? Everything goes out of what. Your kidney and liver get overworked, your brain decreases in functionality, and your emotions feel out of control.

#2. Artificial Sweeteners:

Aspartame, the common ingredient found in products like diet soda, blocks the production of serotonin. That can lead to headaches, insomnia mood swings, among other issues.

#3. Caffeine:

Even a modest amount of caffeine can excavate your anxiety and even contribute to depression. One study found that moderate and high coffee drinkers scored higher on the depression scale among healthy college students than others. Let's also not forget the disruptive effect that caffeine has on sleep. And if you have disturbed sleep, I can assure you, anxiety levels will skyrocket. If you want to aid your healing, this is something you need to avoid at all costs. And I don't just mean coffee. Consider eliminating energy drinks and soda as they too contain plenty of caffeine.

#4. Hydrogenated oil:

Think of fried chicken, fried cheese sticks, fried calamari, french fries, and basically any fried junk food that you usually fall back on when you feel overwhelmed by emotions. Unfortunately, eating this kind of food actually makes things worse in the long run. Saturated fats like the ones found in deli meats, high-fat dairy, and butter can create a lot of damage to your body if they clog your arteries and impede proper blood flow to the brain. I know this sounds super harsh, but the reality is, eating deep-fried foods digs you deeper into anxiety and other mental health disorders.

#5. High sodium foods:

Remember how experts touted fat-free foods as the go-to solution for weight loss? It turns out many of the products endorsed as fat-free contain high levels of sodium. All that extra salt is actually bad for your emotions because it disrupts aspects of your neurological system. Not only can this mess with your mental health, but it can also mess with your immune system response and create an experience of fatigue, bloating, and fluid retention. Foods with high sodium include savory snacks like pretzels, crackers, popcorn and chips, burritos and tacos, cheese, chicken, cold cuts and cured meats, eggs, omelets, and pizza.

#6. Processed foods:

Want to know the perfect storm when it comes to messing up your physical and mental health? Processed foods. They're high in sodium and pave the way for an inflammatory response in the body. An article in Psychiatric Times shared that inflammation has a direct effect on the brain and behavior. It can negatively affect the areas of the brain responsible for motivation and motor activity and the areas that control anxiety and alarm. Before you get disheartened, let me state that you don't need to cut out all processed foods. Examples of processed foods that experts agree can work for someone looking to eat healthier include yogurt, sauerkraut, chickpeas, canned beans, granola, veggie burgers, unsweetened almond milk, organic jelly, fortified cereals, freeze-dried fruit, pickles, and dark chocolate.

9 BEST FOODS FOR REDUCING ANXIETY:

#1. Fatty Fish: Salmon, mackerel, sardines, trout, and herring are among the top favorite fatty fish that should become part of your diet as they are rich in omega-3. Why does omega-3 matter? There's plenty of evidence that links this fatty acid to improved cognitive function and mental health. Omega 3 rich foods that contain alpha-linolenic acid (ALA) provide two important fatty acids, namely: eicosapentaenoic acid (EPA) and docosahexaenoic acid (DHA). Both EPA and DHA regulate neurotransmitters, reduce inflammation and promote healthy brain function. A small study on twenty-four people with substance abuse problems found that the EPA and DHA supplementation reduced anxiety levels. This isn't conclusive research, but it should be enough to convince you of the great benefits that await you. Please note that omega-3 is not identical to omega-6, so don't substitute one for the other. With omega-6, you should only take it in small, moderate quantities.

#2. Pumpkin seeds: A study carried out on 100 female high school students found that zinc deficiency may negatively affect mood. That's why pumpkin seeds are great for your diet. Pumpkin seeds are an excellent source of potassium which helps regulate electrolyte balance and manage blood pressure. It also contains Zinc, which is essential for brain and development, all of which help reduce stress and anxiety symptoms.

#3. Dark chocolate: For most people, dark chocolate's bitter flavor profile is off-putting, but most research indicates it's worth getting used to having a bit of dark chocolate frequently. A 2019 survey-based study published in the journal Depression & Anxiety suggests that people who eat dark chocolate often are less likely to report depressive symptoms. Although depression isn't the same as anxiety, the two share similarities and often go hand in hand. This research is far from conclusive, but I'd say it's worth a try. Consider adding small amounts to your morning cereal or tea.

#4. Turmeric: This is a spice commonly used in India and Southeast Asia. Turmeric contains an active ingredient called curcumin, which has properties that lower anxiety due to its anti-inflammatory properties. One study found that an increase of curcumin in the diet also increased DHA and reduced anxiety. If you're not a fan of pungent spices, don't worry, turmeric has a minimal flavor and can be added to almost any food as well as smoothies.

#5. Yogurt: Go for plain greek yogurt as much as possible, especially the one with at least five strains of active culture and rich in probiotics. The right kind of yogurt is said to be great for alleviating stress and stabilizing your mood.

#6. Kiwi: One of my favorite fruits of all time and apparently promoted by experts as an excellent fruit for reducing stress and anxiety. Studies indicate that the combination of vitamins C and E plus folate may help reduce oxidative stress. It may also help in the production of serotonin in your brain, which will promote a sense of well-being and happiness. Besides, have you seen how beautiful and colorful kiwis are on the inside? Instant mood booster if it's on your breakfast bowl.

#7. Chamomile: A great routine to add to your nighttime ritual is winding up your day with a nice cup of warm, soothing chamomile tea. A 2016 clinical trial with results published in the journal phytomedicine suggests that those who drank tea over a long-term period significantly reduced severe GAD (generalized anxiety disorder) symptoms. Perhaps it's linked to the fact that it enhances your sleepiness, ensuring you get good quality sleep which, as we know, directly impacts mental health, especially anxiety.

#8. Green tea: Are you a fan of herbal tea? More specifically, green tea? If not, it's time to stock up. Green tea contains an amino acid called theanine which has anti-anxiety and calming effects. Some experts claim it increases the production of serotonin and dopamine. This can be an excellent substitute for coffee, soda, or even alcohol.

#9. Avocado: There's no doubt that when it comes to avocado, you can't have too much of this superfood. It's packed with all kinds of excellent nutrients, including vitamin B6 and magnesium, which help with serotonin production. You can find lots of avocado-based recipes for breakfast, lunch, and dinner on YouTube and Google.

MOVING YOUR BODY HELPS INCREASE HAPPY HORMONES

You've heard me talk about diet and the importance of eating the right food because food affects your mental state just as much as it affects your physical condition. Now let's add another critical component to your recovery plan: exercise.

Most people only value exercise when they need to lose a few pounds before beach season kicks in. But if you want to transform your life and enjoy holistic health, some form of regular exercising will have to become your new norm. Research has found that your diet, fitness level, and the amount of stress you're exposed to directly influence your panic disorder and anxiety. By exercising your body regularly, you can help reduce anxiety and even the frequency and intensity of panic attacks. I also find exercise to be an excellent way for me to release mental and physical tension. Why does exercise work?

- Because exercise releases feel-good endorphins and other natural brain chemicals that enhance your sense of wellbeing.
- While exercising, you actually take your mind off worrisome thoughts and emotions, which cuts that cycle of negative thinking.
- It's a great coping strategy. Doing something positive to distract yourself when having a tough day (like Yoga, Pilates, Endurance training, or cross-training) is much better than binge-eating or alcohol. It gives you a win-win situation where you come out feeling good, help your body get fit, and keeps intrusive thoughts at bay.
- Exercise also increases your confidence levels. Think about it. Doesn't it feel good to set a goal of working out daily for 20 minutes and then actually showing yourself that you can commit and get it done?

I often have forced myself to start my workout routine, and it felt almost impossible to get my body moving. Still, fifteen minutes into it, I felt so glad that I began the workout. By the time the week was over, I was so proud to see tick marks of success on my journal, demonstrating I was still on my workout streak. It made me feel like I can do anything else I set my mind to. These mini-goals are great for boosting confidence. And of course, there's the added bonus of having a better-shaped body, which makes us feel good.

Do you need to join a gym or jog to work out your body?

You absolutely don't need a gym membership or train with weights or even jog outdoors if none of these things apply to you. A gym membership is great for the person who needs that feeling of community and support, and social interaction. But if you feel better working out in the comfort of your apartment, then, by all means, do that!

If you're a complete beginner, you could start with something as simple as regular power walks, light jogging outdoors, playing football, basketball, or any other fitness activity that gets your heart pumping and your body sweating. If none of these appeals to you, consider Pilates, power yoga, Zumba, kickboxing, or Latin dance lessons.

The most important thing is that you enjoy the activity you're doing and create your own plan of action that you can stick to.

What are the best anti-anxiety workouts?

- Running
- Power walks
- Dancing
- Tennis

- Swimming
- Biking
- Yoga

TOP FOUR EXERCISES YOU CAN TRY AT HOME

#1: Tai Chi:

This is a soft martial art that includes fluid movements along with core control. You will focus on posture, breathing, and visualization in this workout, making it great for de-stressing and feeling rooted in your body.

#2: High-Intensity home workout:

When you go on YouTube, you can find dozens of free high-intensity workout routines that you can do from the comfort of your bedroom or living area. An article from Science Daily shares some interesting findings on the effect of high-intensity exercises in relation to reducing anxiety. A new study by researchers at the University of Missouri-Columbia shows that relatively high-intensity training is superior in reducing stress and anxiety. Moreover, the researchers found that high-intensity exercise primarily benefits women. The older you are, the more you'll notice the positive impact on your physical and mental state (sourced from Sciencedaily.com "High-Intensity Exercise Best Way To Reduce Anxiety, University of Missouri Study Finds).

So, if Tai chi is a bit too chilled for you, or if you just want to mix things up a bit, try doing high-intensity workouts a few times a week.

#3: Aerobics:

Regular aerobic exercising (swimming, cycling, running) is associated with better psychological health. According to recent studies, whether it's a single session or a long-term program for aerobics exercises, you can improve your psychological state. How long is enough to reap some rewards of aerobic exercises? As little as ten minutes but experts encourage you to consistently stick to the exercise regimen for at least 10 weeks for maximum benefit. YouTube is filled with tons of free aerobics workouts that you can follow along. Check out HASfit on YouTube for free workouts and workout programs if you're confused about where to start. All you need is a mat for comfort and a stretch band. If you enjoy indoor running, swimming, or cycling, consider joining a club near you to make it easy for you to do it daily.

#4: Yoga:

This list wouldn't be complete without some yoga which has become the go-to exercise for people wanting to channel their inner Zen and at the same time burn some calories. The nature of yoga focused on deep breathing, reconnecting with your body, and getting grounded within yourself. This is great for someone suffering from anxiety because it enables you to tap into your inner strength and to show yourself that you have the power to do amazing things with your body. And if you can change your body, surely you can change your thoughts. The fact is yoga works every single time! Unless you quit on yourself.

Studies show that yoga classes can help you reduce anxiety, anger, depression, and even neurotic symptoms. According to a Harvard

Medical School Article (Yoga for anxiety and depression), research suggests that yoga modulates stress response systems. That, in turn, decreases psychological arousal (e.g., reducing the heart rate, lowering blood pressure, and easing respiration). Substantial evidence is building up to demonstrate that yoga practice is a relatively low-risk, high-yield approach to improving overall health. And the best part is it's easy to do, and you can find free yoga sessions online or join a virtual or physical yoga class. All you need is a yoga mat and a nice set of lungs for intentional breathing!

Bonus:

Once you decide what exercises you will commit to, create a customized plan that's easy to follow. Don't overcomplicate things and keep your workout program as simple and as enjoyable as you possibly can. Be flexible with the program. If you usually get bored quickly, create a variety of exercises that you can keep changing up week after week so you can stick to your workout goals. Make your goals attainable and celebrate the small wins. Instead of striving for perfection, focus on progress and excellence. If you stop during an exercise or don't complete a set in any workout, don't assume that means failure. Instead, recognize that you are on a journey that won't always be easy. The most important thing is that you pick yourself up and go at it again with vigor and enthusiasm, trusting that each move is getting you closer to that healthy version of yourself.

A GOOD NIGHT'S SLEEP DOES MORE THAN YOU THINK

By now, you may have realized we are establishing the lifestyle changes that will enable you to transform your health and life. These things all build upon each other. Without the right nutrition, you won't have the energy or stamina to workout daily. And without sleep, it doesn't matter how good your diet is or how much you kill yourself in the gym; it will all fall apart. Poor sleep directly impacts your mental health. You cannot reduce or heal anxiety disorders without proper sleep. Your mood, cognitive functions, and overall health depend on you to work appropriately. So, one of the first things you need to work on (I mean starting tonight) is to adjust your sleeping habits. You need restorative sleep to maintain a balanced brain. Sleep quality and length do matter; let no one tell you differently. Research shows that sleep-deprived individuals have a stronger tendency to classify neutral images as negative. That means ordinary experiences that you encounter on a daily basis will seem more menacing and contribute to your anxiety.

Falling asleep and getting good quality sleep is often a challenge when battling anxiety disorders. So, what can you do?

#1: Avoid stimulants later in the day:

If you can cut out all stimulants, that would be the best solution, but I know it might be difficult for some. So instead, I want you to have a limit after which you will consume no stimulants. I recommend setting a curfew for yourself depending on your lifestyle and work schedule but roughly six to eight hours before bedtime. So, if your bedtime is 10pm, then you shouldn't consume any stimulants after 4 pm latest.

#2: Try this 3-minute relaxation technique:

Lie flat and comfortably on your bed. Focus your attention on your breathing. Take a few deep breaths, exhaling slowly. Mentally scan your body. Take notice of any areas that feel tense and cramped. Gently loosen them. Let go of as much tension as you can. Rotate your head in a gentle and smooth circular motion once or twice if it feels good. Roll your shoulders forward and backward several times. Let all of your muscles completely relax. Recall a pleasant thought, event, or place. It can be as recent as today or something that happened in the past. Notice how your body feels as you soak in this good memory. Take deep breaths and exhale slowly.

#3: Create an ideal sleep environment:

That includes ensuring your smartphone and any technology that distracts you are out of reach. Try keeping your phone as far away from your sleeping area as possible. It's also important to shut out all light from your bedroom. This is especially useful if you have trouble falling asleep. Also, remember to minimize noise and keep the room temperature cool enough to be under a blanket. Suppose there's a particular scent that helps you relax or fall asleep. In that case, you can spray it or light a candle as you get ready for bed so it can aid you in this relaxation and sleeping process.

#4: Create a calming sleep routine:

It's just as important to have a routine for your bedtime as it is in the morning because it helps you wind down and fall asleep faster. Certain activities are too stimulating and bad for your anxiety when done too close to your bedtime. This includes social media browsing, alcohol and coffee consumption, and even high-intensity workouts. Although exercise is good for you, doing it just before bed will make it hard to fall asleep.

Although there's no perfect sleep routine, a few things you may want to consider include:

a. setting the alarm sixty minutes before bedtime to indicate to your brain that it's time to unwind and let go of a hectic day. Once that alarm goes off, don't snooze or ignore it. Do not keep binge-watching television or chatting with friends. Instead, move into your personalized unwind routine.

b. Make yourself some relaxing herbal tea like chamomile and sit with a book for a few minutes or listen to some soothing music.

c. Guided meditation for relaxation and sleep can be great at this point if that resonates.

d. Wash up before bed. If you like baths or a hot shower before sleeping, you can do that. Otherwise, some dental hygiene and a gentle facewash are sufficient. As you wash up, practice some mindfulness and notice the sensation of your teeth as you brush and how the water feels in your hands and face.

e. Set the mood in your bedroom. Whether you have a partner or not, it's good to select the right mood, including dim lighting and cool temperature, to send the signal to your body that you're ready for sleep.

f. Do you like essential oils and aromatherapy? Then add fragrances like lavender and cedarwood to your routine by placing a diffuser in your bedroom or using a few drops of essential oil on your pillow before bed. If you like baths, consider scenting it with a few drops of your favorite essential oil.

g. Think peaceful thoughts. Instead of fixating on worrisome thoughts of things that haven't yet happened or things that have already passed, try focusing on something that makes you feel good. This would be an excellent time to practice some evening gratitude, visualizing a restful scene where you would enjoy falling asleep and basically using your imagination to aid you into relaxation instead of allowing it to run wild. You need to tame your mind and teach your imagination to go where you want it to go, especially in the evening. Do you enjoy quiet beaches? Why not visualize yourself walking barefoot on a beautiful beach with waves brushing against the shore and the sand on your feet. Practice breathing slowly and peacefully as you relax in this chosen environment.

h. Do a body scan as soon as you hit the bed. Once you get into bed, your brain will probably start drifting and thinking about a million things. Bring it to your body and do a body scan as you relax your muscles. Here's a simple exercise to try. Slowly tense one group of muscles. Hold the tension to the count of five, then release slowly as you exhale. Relax to the count of ten, then move to the next muscle group. Begin from the toes all the way up to your head, one muscle group at a time, and think of nothing else.

i. Read something spiritually uplifting and joyful. Now is not the time to read the news or thriller novels. You don't want to stimulate your brain or nervous system, so instead, I encourage you to find something spiritual, philosophical, or comical to read. If you are a person of faith, then read a passage from the Bible. If you enjoy fairytales, comics or jokes, then read that and if you enjoy ancient thinkers, then read a page from Aristotle if that's your thing.

What happens when you just can't sleep no matter what you try?

On those nights when nothing works, don't force it. Practice acceptance. Use the power of validation and positive self-talk to make this experience okay too. Instead of getting upset over the fact that you've been lying there for three hours and nothing happened, you can say to yourself, "I'm still awake now, but sooner or later, I will have to fall asleep. Even if it's not this night, the fact that I will be a little tired in the morning means I'll probably fall asleep right away tomorrow night." One thing I would advise when it comes to insomnia, I find it better to wake up and do some quiet activity instead of lying there in frustration. I will pick a book and read if it's too late or too early in the morning to do something else.

CUT DOWN THE STRESSORS!

Stress and anxiety go hand in hand, but they aren't the same. Stress is any strain on your brain or physical body. Since all biological experiences impact your psychology, a stressed-out body or brain will mess with your mental health. While treating anxiety and panic attacks, stress can make the process more difficult, especially if you have a stressful lifestyle. When combined, stress and anxiety can make your life feel like a living hell. So, we need to do everything possible to reduce, manage or, if possible, eliminate the things that cause you to get stressed.

Of course, if you tell me you hate your boss and your job and that it's the number one cause for stress in your life right now, that's a doozy. It's not exactly smart to eliminate this stress by quitting your job because you open up a host of reasons to be anxious and fearful, like facing unemployment, running out of rent money, etc. So, there are some cases where you need to exercise stress management. One thing you can do to manage work stress is to implement the changes already discussed, i.e., get a healthy diet, limit caffeine and alcohol, exercise, meditate, and get enough sleep. But sometimes, your anxiety is triggered while at work, even if you're practicing this new lifestyle shift. In that case, you need a way out. Here are a few things you can instantly do at work to bring your stress levels down.

#1. Listen to your favorite song:

There's always that one song that can take you from dystopia to utopia in a matter of minutes. That song should always be on your smartphone for those days when everyone at work seems to push your buttons. Step away from the room for a few minutes, find some-where with some fresh air (a terrace, the rooftop, outside the office building), and plug-in your earphones for a few minutes. Breathe deeply, dance to the beat, sing aloud if it's safe, and just allow yourself to be elsewhere for those three minutes. Playing music has a positive effect on the brain and body. It can lower blood pressure, reduce cortisol, and if you pick the right jam, it will fill you with boundless joy and happiness in no time.

#2: Do some belly breathing:

Breathing from your diaphragm can help reduce the amount of work your body needs to do to breathe. At work, you can do this by sitting in a comfortable chair with your head, neck and shoulders relaxed and your knees bent. Put one hand under your rib cage and one hand over your heart. Inhale and exhale through your nose, noticing how or if your stomach and chest move as you breathe. Focus on breathing more through your belly instead of your chest. Notice the movement (the rise and fall of your abdomen) and the corresponding sensations within your body. Try to keep your chest as still as possible for this type of breathing. You can do this for as little as five minutes, and you will feel the full effect if you go up to ten minutes.

#3: Chew gum:

This is an easy and quick fix that can help calm you down in almost any situation, whether at work or home. One study showed that people who chew gum had a greater sense of wellbeing and lower stress levels. This might be due to the fact that chewing gum causes brain waves similar to those of relaxed people, and it promotes blood flow to the brain.

#4: Learn to say no:

Sometimes the thing causing you to stress is out of your control, or worse still, it's unnecessary added pressure. If you like people-pleasing, it will be hard to reduce your anxiety because you'll keep piling on things to do for others, making your life more difficult. If you find yourself taking on more than you can handle, it's time to learn how to say no. Be selective about what you take on, and remember, no is a full sentence. You don't have to justify yourself or feel guilty, especially when you already know you have many responsibilities. Learning to say no can significantly reduce or help you manage your stress levels.

8

BEDTIME: MORE THAN CREATING A ROUTINE

According to Harvard Medical School, sleep difficulties affect more than 50% of adult patients with a generalized anxiety disorder. It will impact teenagers and children as well. One sleep laboratory study found that youngsters with an anxiety disorder took longer to fall asleep and slept less deeply when compared with a control group of healthy children. Insomnia is also considered a risk factor for developing an anxiety disorder and may even prevent recovery. So, if you thought sleep was a trivial matter or that creating calming sleep routines was just nice to have, think again. In this chapter, I want to awaken you to the benefits of getting proper rest and sell you on the fact that you need to do everything in your power to improve your current sleep pattern. Let's start with some simple facts about how sleeping well keeps you healthy.

SLEEP AND ITS HOLISTIC BOOST TO YOUR HEALTH

Research has shown that sleep is just as important as eating and exercise for anyone who wants to enjoy a healthy, vibrant lifestyle. Poor sleep is linked to increased body weight, depression, increased inflammation, low concentration levels, mood disorders, low productivity levels, increased stress, and increased risk of heart disease and stroke. What's more, even a small loss of sleep has been shown to impair immune function.

In a sizeable 2-week study that monitored the development of the common cold (participants were given nasal drops with the cold virus). The study found that those who slept less than 7 hours were almost three times more likely to develop a cold than those who slept 8 hours or more. So, sleep runs deeper than just aiding in your mental health. Consider for a moment how often you get colds. If you frequently fall sick, switching up your sleep time and getting adequate hours for your body type can help, especially during the colder months. Besides all these side effects of being sleep deprived, there are many other ways your body will benefit from good sleep.

Sharper brain and optimum cognitive functioning:

When operating with little to no sleep, you'll struggle to focus, learn, or recall details. Why? Because sleep plays a big part in both learning and memory. Without proper sleep, taking in new information is very troublesome. Your reflexes also slow down when sleep-deprived, so by increasing sleep time, you get to improve how your brain and body function and assimilates information.

Stronger immune system:

The immune system is a complex network that's spread out throughout your body. It provides multiple lines of defense against illness. When functioning optimally, the immune system will maintain that delicate balance needed to keep you feeling and looking healthy. When a threat or injury arises, it triggers inflammation, fatigue, fever, and pain. We need the immune system to be strong enough to fight any and all potential threats. We also need it to be well regulated so that the body isn't always in attack mode, as that isn't ideal either. That's where sleep comes in.

Getting sufficient hours of high-quality sleep enables your body to create the right atmosphere for a well-balanced immune system that is efficient, responsive when needed, and less prone to allergic reactions. As the body sleeps, certain components of the immune system get revved up. For example, there's an increased production of cytokines associated with inflammation. This activity appears to be driven both by sleep and circadian rhythm (the body's 24-hour internal clock).

Although experts aren't entirely sure why the immune system works best during sleep time, it is believed that this system works best when physical and mental performance are at a minimum. As breathing and muscle activity slows down, there's more energy for the immune system to perform its tasks. Also, we know that melatonin (a sleep-promoting hormone) is adept at counteracting the stress that can come from inflammation during sleep.

Mood booster:

Another benefit of sleep is natural emotion regulation which also boosts your mood. It stabilizes your emotions and makes it easier for you to handle and process your feelings. If something unpleasant or unexpected happens, you're more likely to remain calm and optimistic when you're well-rested.

BEDTIME ROUTINE TO HELP YOU GET A GOOD NIGHT'S SLEEP

In the previous chapter, you learned that a good night's sleep can do wonders for your mental health. That's why I emphasized the importance of creating a calming sleep routine. In case you are wondering where to begin or what specific things you can do to promote high-quality sleep, here are more tips proven to work.

Reduce blue light exposure after sunset:

You have an internal clock often referred to as the circadian rhythm, which regulates hormones like melatonin. Melatonin is essential in helping you relax and get deep sleep. Blue light, usually found in electronic devices like smartphones and computers, is the worst for the emission of this type of light. It tricks your brain into thinking it's still daytime. And unfortunately, that inhibits your ability to feel sleepy. You can do a few things if you must use these gadgets, including installing an app that blocks blue light on your smartphone and laptop. You can also wear glasses that block blue light. Since television and bright lights also contribute to the delay of melatonin release, you may want to stop watching TV and turn off bright lights two hours before bedtime.

Create a set time to sleep and wake up:

Consistency with your sleep and waking times can help you align with your circadian rhythm and promote better quality sleep. Irregular sleep patterns lead to poor sleep and confuse your circadian rhythm. In fact, it's not enough to go to bed early some days and later on others. The idea that you can sleep late on weekends only is actually bad for your health. If possible, try to wake up naturally at a similar time every day that aligns with your lifestyle. You don't need to be an early bird. What you need is to understand your best wake-up time and maintain it.

Avoid late-night meals:

Eating late at night may negatively impact your sleep and the natural release of HGH and melatonin. That's not to say you should never snack at night. A study found that a high carb meal eaten four hours before bed helped people sleep faster, while another discovered that a low carb diet also improved sleep. So, what does that mean for you? That there's no right or wrong. Find what works best for your body, and you will know based on how well you sleep. As a general rule of thumb, late-night snacking should be as light on your digestive system as possible, and there shouldn't be any stimulants consumed in the process.

Don't drink liquids before bed:

Hydrating with plenty of water throughout the day is terrific. But you don't want to wait till bedtime to gobble down the last six glasses that you missed during the day. Why? Because that interrupted sleep that will ensue (thanks to the frequent peeing that will be involved) will affect sleep quality.

Everyone is different, so some people might be okay with a glass or two of water just before jumping into bed. Maybe even a few cups of herbal tea half an hour before bed won't create any interference, but if you realize you pee a lot, I suggest no drinks one to two hours before sleep time. You should also pee right before jumping into bed to reduce the chance of waking up in the middle of the night.

WOULD YOUR ROOM SET UP AFFECT THE WAY YOU SLEEP?

The answer is absolutely yes. Various studies indicate that external noise, often from traffic, can cause poor sleep and long-term health issues. One study on women's bedroom environment showed that 50% of the participants noticed improved sleep quality when noise and light diminished. As such, it's imperative to make some adjustments to the current state of your sleeping quarters.

A great place to start is with your curtains, the lighting system, and the room temperature. These are simple, quick fixes you can do regardless of your location, and they will impact your sleep. See if you can minimize external noise and light. Get some dimly lit lampshades instead of the bright overhead bedroom lights. Make sure your bedroom is as quiet, relaxing, and clean as it can be. I have a friend who completely blocked out the windows in his bedroom by covering them up with wooden blocks. That kept out all light and noise, so even though he lives in a rather noisy apartment building, his bedroom is completely peaceful and Zen-like.

Not a fan of completely darkening your room?

Consider purchasing room-darkening blinds, shades, or drapes that allow you to go totally dark in the evening but still have some sunshine during the day.

CONTROL YOURSELF IN THE THINGS TO DO AND NOT TO DO IN BED

Given how tricky this topic of sleep is for us, we need to increase our discipline around bedtime rituals and get honest about what we can and cannot control. What happens in the bedroom is entirely under your control. The neighbors, streetcars, or whatever else happens outside your home will never be in your control, so if you get frustrated by the noisy neighbors who seem to enjoy cranking on the music till the wee hours of the night in the middle of the week, consider what you can do in your sleeping space to eliminate more of that noise.

Take a moment not to consider the quality and quantity of your sleep. But how easy has it been for you to fall asleep in the last few months? Do you often wake up in the middle of the night and struggle to fall back asleep? Are there any distractions in your room that might be affecting your sleep?

What you want to eliminate from the bedroom:

Don't feed in bed:

If you can avoid eating anything before bed, that is ideal. But suppose you had a long day and got home late, so you need a snack before jumping into bed. In that case, eat standing by the kitchen counter and make sure it isn't something fatty. Whole grain bread with some peanut butter spread ought to ease those hunger pangs and enable you to sleep well. What you must never do is carry your food to the bedroom. Not only is this poor hygiene because you're likely to start attracting all kinds of bugs into your bed, but it's also a very unhealthy habit to get into. All food should be left in the living quarters unless there's a medical reason causing you to feed in bed.

The television:

If your television is in your bedroom, it's time to exile it to the living room. Watching some tv, whether it's comedy or horror, has adverse effects on your sleep. Sleep specialist W. Christopher Winter, MD, says that the glowy effect of the screen actually stimulates our brain and inhibits the secretion of melatonin. Regardless of how comforting you find watching an episode of *Friends* before sleeping, stop watching an hour before sleep and do it elsewhere - not in the bedroom.

Avoid having intensely negative discussions in the bedroom:

For many married couples of those in a committed relationship, the only chance for connecting with your loved one is at the end of the busy day (more specifically in bed). If there's a pending discussion, a disagreement, or something intense that must be discussed, I urge you to pause it until the next morning. If it cannot wait, then have a discussion before both of you are lying in bed trying to fall asleep. Do not engage in negative talk, trying to hash things out right before sleep. Instead, I want you to make your bedroom area a sanctuary. The place where only positive vibes are allowed. Intimacy, romance, cuddling, and encouragement should be the only activities going on under the sheets. All else should be off-limits once you get under the sheets. Besides, most arguments dissipate when a couple "sleeps on it" because we all tend to be more rational and calmer in the morning.

Don't sleep with the family pet:

Yes, I know how much you love your pet and how comforting it is to have it lying next to you. But suppose you're struggling with insomnia or severe sleep deprivation. In that case, you really want to consider giving your pet a new bed. Pets can sometimes make it hard for us to sleep because they can create sleep disruption as they move, twitch, and breathe. We can find ourselves waking up several times in one night, which is really bad for recovery. You don't necessarily need to get them out of the bedroom but just let them sleep in their own space so you can have more freedom to get a full night's sleep.

The last tip I want to give that is entirely within your control is to train yourself into the habit of using the bedroom purely for sleep and intimacy. Condition your brain to refuse anything else. That includes working on your laptop while in bed, browsing Instagram and Facebook, or even talking on the phone. When you get under the sheets, it should be either to sleep, which should happen within that first half-hour or to make love with your partner, which will ultimately enable you to relax and sleep. This is all part of your sleep hygiene. By including the tips shared in your evening routine, you are more likely to see significant changes in your sleep quality and quantity.

9

THE WILDLY EFFECTIVE, YET SURPRISINGLY SIMPLE, METHOD FOR STOPPING PANIC ATTACKS IN THEIR TRACKS (AND WAYS TO REDUCE THEIR FREQUENCY!)

Don't panic! How many times have you heard that? If only it were that easy. Panic attacks suck, but you know what sucks even more? That feeling of powerlessness, knowing that you can't control or stop anything. Now, I know everyone experiences their own version of panic attack disorders, but what if you could learn some simple and healthy coping techniques that could actually help you stop the attacks before they cause any significant damage?

Plan an Escape Route and Develop Coping Techniques Before Panic Attacks:

Trying to control a panic attack or avoid it entirely before recovery is at 100% is futile, in my opinion. In fact, I think even after your treatment and recovery, you should never worry about not getting another attack. Instead, focus on healthy strategies to immediately help you alleviate an attack's symptoms long before maturity.

A metaphor I like to use is this: If you're running a race carrying a boiled egg on a small spoon that must get to the finish line, I wouldn't worry so much about dropping the egg. Instead, I would focus on what needs to happen so that whenever the egg drops, I can easily pick it up without damaging it and continue my race to the end.

The same is true for your healing and overall mental wellbeing. You don't have to be perfect to declare yourself healed. But you do need to know exactly what to do as soon as the first sign of an anxiety or panic attack rears its ugly head. That demands a carefully thought out plan which includes healthy coping mechanisms.

KNOW YOURSELF AND YOUR TRIGGERS:

The more you know yourself and how you react to certain stimuli or situations, the easier it becomes to identify those triggers. For example, you might realize that your morning rush often generates a lot of anxiety. What does that tell you? The morning ritual has to be transformed into something that produces calm and ease. The more control you have with your morning, the less likely you will spiral downward and activate an attack. By integrating things like mindfulness meditation, yoga, journaling, and so on into your morning routine, you will see that internal shift that will bring out the desired change in your mental state.

Another thing you need to do is learn to recognize your symptoms. That involves knowing how your body feels and identifying your thought processes as anxiety begins to build. So, think for a moment about the sensations and biological cues that typically overwhelm your system right as the stress gains momentum. Do you usually start shaking, or does your stomach fill up with butterflies? Perhaps for you, it's a tightening on your stomach and a sense of "lack of air" as your breath quickens and shortens. It's very possible that even before the physical symptoms, there are psychological warning signs that pop up, like intrusive thoughts which trigger that feeling of nervousness. The more you can catch any of these psychological and biological signals, the easier it becomes to end the anxiety before it blows up into an actual attack.

Now I want to share some healthy coping strategies that you will need to practice when in a relaxed state. I suggest doing them daily so they can stick and become the natural impulse when you get triggered.

Deep breathing:

As soon as those overwhelming emotions kick in, the first step should be to distance yourself from that environment. You don't need to make any drastic physical changes, but you need to distance yourself mentally, and the best way to do that is through deep breathing.

Take long, deep breaths and mentally count to ten (backwards). Inhale through the nose and out through the mouth. If you lose count, start again from ten moving toward one. That will distract you from the heat of the moment, reconnect you to your breath (which is a powerful anchoring technique). By pumping more blood into the brain, you'll tend to feel less tense and more balanced.

Sometimes, the breathwork isn't enough to pause the panic attack, so try one of the other techniques.

Get grounded:

A great grounding technique is about tuning into yourself and finding a stabilizing point. See if you can close your eyes for five seconds, then reopen and connect with 4 things that you can see in that immediate surrounding. Can you mentally name the 4 objects or something that you see? Great. Next, I want you to touch 3 things (a table, the wall, a curtain, or anything else), smell two things, and taste 1 thing in your immediate vicinity. If you happen to be at your cubicle, then touch the surfaces next to you, including your own body parts, open up a book and smell that and just focus on tasting the insides of your mouth. Of course, I prefer you go outside for more variety but do the best where you are under current circumstances. What matters in this grounding exercise is that you force your mind to connect with your external senses.

Ice yourself:

Ice packs work for many people, so consider keeping some ice packs in the freezer, especially if you get those nighttime panic attacks. A friend of mine usually has two small and two big ice packs ready to go. When he feels panic coming, he puts the small ones in his hands and the large ones either on his lower back or belly. When he has difficulty breathing, he will usually grab an ice pack and rub it from the middle of his chest down to the bottom of his belly very slowly until his heart rate starts to mellow. You might want to try this out as well.

Carry some lavender essential oil or a scented handkerchief:

Lavender is considered a powerful soothing agent. Sometimes, it might be all you need to stop growing anxiety. Many studies show that lavender can help relieve stress. If you get the oil, try holding it under your nose and inhaling gently or dabbing a little onto your handkerchief to smell. The best kind is the natural essential oil, as that is the safest to inhale. You can also apply a little on your wrists, almost like perfume, rub them together and inhale throughout the day as needed.

Not a fan of lavender? Try out chamomile, lemon, orange, or bergamot and see if they work for you

Repeat a mantra:

A mantra is a word, phrase, or sound that you repeat until you gain some sense of calmness and focus. Internally repeating a mantra can really help you put a stop to an oncoming panic attack. It doesn't have to be something grandiose as long as the mantra resonates with you deeply. If you're a person of faith, you could quote a verse from the Bible or even say a simple phrase like "This too shall pass." If you enjoy Sanskrit mantras, you could find one that makes you feel good such as "Sat. Chit. Ananda."

The main objective is to gently repeat the mantra and to bring all your focus on the feeling generated by that calming, soothing repetition until your physical state slows down and your breathing and muscles relax.

HOW SIMPLE IS THIS SIMPLE METHOD?

Panic attacks usually feel like you're literally choking to death. You may feel like you're hyperventilating or experiencing shortness of breath. The best way to get through an attack is by simply focusing on your breath and doing this simple breathing exercise.

Start by breathing slowly and purposefully to counteract that shallow breathing that's attempting to enhance the attack. If comfortable, place your hands on your belly and fill it with the breath. As you inhale, feel, and connect with this rising sensation as the belly expands. As you exhale, the abdomen will contract inward. Follow this movement and drain it of every bit of air. You could also count each breath. For example, count to four as you inhale, hold for three, then count to four as you exhale. Keep all your focus here. Center yourself in this movement and focus on that slow inhale and slow exhale. Do this until you feel a shift and your body and mind feel soothed. It's a simple exercise, but there is great power in mindfulness breathing. If you can stay in it for as little as seven minutes without allowing yourself to drift anywhere else, you will bring yourself back to a calm state and chase away that attack naturally.

∾

7 ADDITIONAL SIMPLE TIPS TO REDUCE YOUR ANXIETY (AND PANIC ATTACK) WHENEVER IT FLARES UP, NO MATTER WHERE YOU ARE

#1: Close your eyes:

Sometimes the panic attack or anxiety is exacerbated by the stimuli in your environment, making it harder for you to focus on your breath, so consider closing your eyes if it's safe enough. Allow those external stimuli to fade into the distance and bring your attention back to the breath. Then follow the simple breathing technique shared earlier.

#2: Engage in light exercise:

This may not apply to all situations, but if you generally enjoy exercising, it might be good to engage in some light workout as you feel the anxiety building. Pause what you're doing and take a ten-minute power walk, skip rope, dance, do some power yoga or bike for a few minutes, allowing your mind to focus entirely on the physical effort you're making and giving your body the chance to break a sweat.

#3: Remind yourself that this is not the end:

Often when we are getting an anxiety attack, we feel like the world is coming to an end or as though it will last forever. When those thoughts start creeping in, remind yourself that this too shall pass.

#4: Focus on an object:

When the mind is racing, it's hard to control your anxiety or even focus on your coping techniques. I like to use an object to curb the distressing signals, feelings, and emotions until I feel centered. I carry around a family heirloom that I use as my object of attention whenever necessary. Still, you can choose any item that captures your interest. It can be a plant in your office, a candle, seashell, a smooth stone, or any object with enough depth to grab your attention. Think about the purpose of the item, the shape, and maybe even its origin.

#5: Switch to a less anxiety-filled task:

Sometimes the easiest way to avoid getting an anxiety attack is to remove yourself from the current task and do something that takes your mind off your worries. It is especially true if you recognize the task at hand is one that triggers your anxiety.

I am not advocating procrastination here. Just give yourself a break and do something enjoyable until your mind returns to a calmer state. Then reframe your perception about the task that's triggering your anxiety. Only when it feels okay do I suggest jumping back into the task with lots of breaks in between.

#6: Fact check your thoughts:

Some, in fact, many of the thoughts that come up when you're about to get an anxiety attack are distorted and harmful to your mental well-being. Consider pausing and doing a self-analysis of the thoughts driving you to believe that something is wrong. You might be surprised to realize that the thoughts are triggering anxiety even though it's unnecessary. For example, if you find yourself thinking, "I'm going to die, "... It's a good idea to question that thought. Ask yourself, "Am I really going to die? Is there a bomb, dangerous animal, or anything in my vicinity that is actually threatening my life?"

I used to be bullied by this thought for almost 2 decades of my life. Eventually, I realized it would show up right before an attack manifested. So, I decided to fact-check it whenever my mind went there. Ultimately, the thought would come. It wouldn't freak me out so much because I had developed this new understanding about myself and how much I fear dying. Then I also learned to make peace with the fact that everyone will die. If mine is today, then I'm at peace with that. But there sure as heck better be an entirely justifiable reason for why I would be thinking that when I'm in a supermarket grocery shopping!

#7: Listen to your favorite song or watch a funny clip:

This works really well for some people, especially if you have a special connection with music or if you've had a childhood program that instantly changes your mental state.

I encourage you to have a playlist at hand that can be your go-to technique as soon as you sense the tension building. Music is known to have many healing properties, so go ahead and give yourself a five-minute music party in your office cubicle and watch the tension melt away.

10

LONG-TERM STRATEGIES TO HELP YOU REDUCE & OVERCOME YOUR ANXIETY ONCE AND FOR ALL, NOT JUST FOR A FEW WEEKS

If you want to truly transform your life and overcome anxiety, you need to play the long game. Techniques and instant fixes are great, but nothing beats having the confidence that you are genuinely healed. That requires making some lifestyle changes, educating yourself on what anxiety is, how it manifests in your life, and what you can do to permanently heal. So far, you've been learning about the facts around this mental disorder. Now you need to personalize that education so you can implement it.

LONG-TERM HEALING STARTS WITH LEARNING:

Do you consider yourself a lifelong learner? If learning has a negative connotation in your life, you will need to shift that belief system because your continued education on mental health and wellbeing will become your saving grace. To understand more about your body and how you function, you will need to educate yourself on how your mind and body work and how your psychological states influence your biological states. Although this book has given you a beginner's crash course, it should not be the end but merely the first step toward further learning. There are many ways to obtain this knowledge. Google is one of the best resources at your fingertips but make sure to learn from trusted websites like mentalhealth.gov, goodtherapy.org or ask your physician for resources and referrals.

Since everyone experiences anxiety in their own unique way, you will need to educate yourself on how your anxiety shows up and what triggers it. Once you can clearly identify both symptoms and triggers, you'll be able to create the right treatment regimen and even identify the right talk therapy should you choose to go down that route. Using your mind to bring back a calm state when anxiety and panic start to show up will require a lot of discipline, so you need to start investing in the necessary resources and develop the practices mentioned earlier. But even with gained knowledge, you might still find yourself completely blanking out whenever it's a severe episode. After all, it can be hard to keep your head straight when your mind and body go into a "death is imminent" state. So, although I want you to use all the other techniques and mindset strategies already explained, here are some specific thoughts you can unleash, especially when panic strikes.

Thought reframes that can help you curb negative thinking.

First, say to yourself, "whatever happens, it's okay. I choose to not feel anxiety. Having the symptom is bad enough. I don't need to add oil to the fire. Been there, done that. I choose not to fear this. And I choose to accept myself and the current situation just as it is."

Second, if the symptom is still persisting, grab your phone and call a friend or therapist. Let them know what's happening. If you have an ongoing treatment regimen that you created for yourself, you can also switch to that. The most important thing is to avoid freaking out, judging yourself harshly, or making yourself feel wrong for feeling as you do.

RELAXATION TECHNIQUES ARE YOUR NEW BEST FRIEND

Relation techniques are great for helping you prevent anxiety and panic attacks. The examples I will be sharing are scientifically proven to slow down your heart rate, lower blood pressure, slow down your breathing, reduce tension, and even boost your confidence. If you also feel like you need to work on your emotions especially intense ones like anger, these exercises may help.

#1: Progressive muscle relaxation:

Experts often refer to this technique as Jacobson relaxation, so don't freak out if you hear that terminology from your doctor. With this technique, you will need to sit or preferably lie down for the best results. What you need is to tighten and relax various muscle groups to stimulate feelings of relaxation and calmness. When doing this exercise, remember to know your boundaries. Do not over-strain your muscles, especially during contraction. Keep your breaths slow and steady as you move from one muscle group to the next. It's best to practice this for a couple of weeks when you're feeling good (you can get into the habit of practicing as soon as you jump into bed and first thing in the morning) so that you can get the hang of it. This technique will be more effective during an anxiety attack only if it has been practiced long enough. There are eight main steps to follow:

- One. Choose a comfortable room with minimal distractions where you can either lie or sit down.
- Two. Start by contracting the muscles in the foot for 5 seconds and releasing the contraction over a ten-second count. Your focus should be to relieve the tension in that particular body part, so notice and feel the muscles relax. If you usually get cramps, splay out the toes instead of curling them inwards. The effect is the same.
- Three. Contract and relax the muscles of the lower legs for the same amount of time.
- Four. Contract and relax the muscles at the hips and buttocks section (this is more impactful if lying down).
- Five. Now do the same on the muscles of the stomach and chest.
- Six. After exercising the torso, contract and relax the shoulders.
- Seven. Next, concentrate on the face muscles. To do this, you can squeeze your eyes shut and clench the jaw for 5 seconds, then slowly release for 10 seconds.
- Eight. The last step is to relax the hands. Make a fist on each hand, hold that contraction for 5 seconds, and then slowly release for 10 seconds.

If you need to use a timer to keep pace with the seconds, that's okay, or you can just count mentally.

Sometimes people use this technique in combination with some of the other methods you'll see below. If that works for you, feel free to experiment.

#2: Deep breathing exercises:

We've emphasized breathing several times in this book but only because of its transformative powers. Use it as a relaxation and meditative technique, and you will experience exhilarating calmness and ease. The whole exercise involves slow deep, and even breaths. That's it! You can do them anytime, anywhere. A particular type of controlled breathing that you can practice today is box breathing.

- One. Start by breathing in through the nose for a count of 2-4 seconds.
- Two. Hold your breath for a count of 2-4 seconds.
- Three. Breath out for a count of 2-4 seconds.
- Four. Hold your breath again for another count of 2-4 seconds.
- Repeat as necessary.

#3: Autogenic training:

Use this relaxation technique to stimulate both psychological and physical calmness. Autogenic training involves slowing and controlling your breath while teaching your body to respond to verbal instructions. For example, you can focus on a particular part of your body and intentionally bring the sensation of warmth and relaxation. You will start to feel a shift and a deep sense of ease coming over you. It's often done with a practitioner, but once you learn the techniques, you can also experiment independently. Here's how.

- One. Sit upright, reclined, or lie down in a position that feels most comfortable for you.
- Two. Begin to introduce verbally some of the sensations you wish to experience and repeat these cues silently. For example, I am completely calm (say it verbally once). My left arm is heavy (repeat this six times). I am completely calm (say it once). My left arm is warm (repeat six times). I am completely calm (say once). My heart beats calmly and regularly (six times). I am completely calm (say once). My heart beats calmly and regularly (six times). I am completely calm (say once). My breathing is calm and regular... it breathes me (six times). I am completely calm (say once).
- Three. Come out of the relaxation by verbally stating, " Arms firm - Breathe deeply - Open eyes." Then follow those instructions.

You can rotate different sensations as you practice this technique. You can induce heaviness, warmth, heart practice (calling attention to the heartbeat, breathing practice (focus on breath), abdominal practice (focus on abdominal sensations), and head practice (focus on the coolness of the forehead).

#4: Biofeedback-assisted relaxation:

Biofeedback-assisted relaxation involves using electronic devices to measure different bodily functions such as skin temperature, pulse rate, or tension in the muscles. The purpose is to help you control or relax a specific part of your body. This technique requires you to attach sensors to the specific part of your body as you relax that muscle group and then monitor and take measurements. This feedback helps you to know which areas to relax and where to focus on most. In most cases, this type of technique is done in a specialist therapy clinic, but you could purchase a portable machine if you want to test it at home. I do, however, caution you to check with your professional healthcare giver before investing in the equipment to ensure they are safe to use and that your body can handle such an experiment.

#5: Guided imagery:

This relaxation technique involves replacing negative or stressful feelings by visualizing pleasant and calming scenarios that trigger corresponding sensations. Suppose you're naturally good at daydreaming or imagining things. In that case, this should be easy to practice, but if all you see when you close your eyes is a never-ending abyss of frightful darkness, then consider either getting some guided meditations or asking your therapist to assist you in guided imagery. Here are three simple steps to test on your own.

- One. Lie down (or sit) in a comfortable position and close your eyes.
- Two. Bring to mind a relaxing environment either from

your memory or something you saw in a movie that you genuinely enjoyed. The best would be to draw from firsthand experience as that would enable you to recall the sensations and elements of that environment. Engage your five senses and notice what you see, smell, hear, taste, and touch.

- Three. Sustain this visualization as long as needed to feel the shift within and remember to take deep breaths as you focus on enhancing the calmness that this exercise brings.

LIFESTYLE CHANGE PLAYS A BIG ROLE IN BATTLING ANXIETY

Deepak Chopra teaches that anxiety is the most common pandemic in our civilization, and it comes about because we anticipate pain in the future. What that implies for us is that the more we train our minds to be present, the easier it will be to manage anxiety. But there's more to this than being present. We also need to deeply assess current habits and lifestyle as these might make our anxiety worse regardless of how much effort we put into being more mindful. Although the standard advice is to seek treatment immediately, let's not overlook the importance of leading a healthy and holistic lifestyle. That also includes having a good work-life balance. Lifestyle includes exercise, nutrition, relationships, time in nature, stress management, recreation, and relaxation, service to others, and spiritual or religious development. We will dive deeper into each of these areas in section three of this book but for now, take a moment to look at these areas as things stand. Do you feel like you're leading a healthy lifestyle? Are all areas thriving? What would you like to shift?

LONG-TERM STRATEGIES COMES WITH LONG-TERM GOALS

If you want your recovery to be enjoyable and successful, you'll need to set some long-term goals that support your healing strategies. Working with a good therapist usually means you also receive guidance on setting goals, but if you're planning on doing this without a therapist, here is an excellent goal-setting formula that will enable you to track progress. It's known as S.M.A.R.T, which is an acronym for **S**pecific **M**easurable **A**ttainable **R**ealistic **T**ime-bound goal setting technique.

To make this practical, think of a desirable objective that you'd like to experience. For example, you might choose to start with a goal of making seven new friends this year if you struggle with social anxiety. That goal is specific (you chose seven friends). It is measurable, attainable, realistic, and time-bound (you decided to do this within 12 months). An unrealistic goal would be never to get a panic attack again. That black and white thinking sets you up for failure. It creates unnecessary pressure because even after healing and recovery, you may periodically experience some symptoms and then handle them before they get out of hand. So instead of creating goals that add pressure and build up your stress in negative ways, use this technique on a goal that you know will thrill you.

First, I want you to identify that goal. What would you like to change concerning your anxiety? Write this in your journal or Google doc and be specific. If you have multiple goals, spread them out so that you have short, medium, and long-term goals that all align. By the way, if you feel a little anxious about the goal, maybe even scared, that's perfectly normal. Right now, is your time to use your imagination productively. Get creative with it, and don't worry about how to do it just yet.

The second step, once the goal/s is clear, is to break it up into digestible chunks. You know you won't be able to go from point A to B in an instant, so we need some mini-milestones along the way. Let me illustrate this with Jenny's story.

Jenny has lived with anxiety since she was sixteen. She always had problems performing well on tests, and despite generally being a good student, panic was the typical reaction during any test or performance check. As she entered the workforce and responsibilities mounted, she experienced everything from a general anxiety disorder when interacting with her manager to full-on panic attacks. The more pressure increased, the more frequent the attacks became.

After seeking some professional guidance, Jenny was finally ready to work on herself and signed up for a talk therapy treatment. But she didn't just leave it at that. Jenny also decided to give herself the feeling of control by creating a S.M.A.R.T goal to ensure she takes back control of her life. The main desirable objective for Jenny was to reduce the frequency and intensity of her attacks. She wanted to get to the point where it doesn't just catch her off guard. So, to make it specific, she went after the frequency and intensity of her panic attack. In order to make this measurable, she decided to track her mood and journal daily. At different points of the day, she would pause for a minute to rate her anxiety level on a scale from 0-10 (with 10 being full-on panic). She committed to these exercises three times a day and diligently recorded the answers on her phone. This was to continue for twelve months at the end of which Jenny wanted to have gradually lowered the frequency down by at least half, which meant, if within the first month she was having an attack twice a week, by the end of the year, she desired it to be once a week. That felt very realistic and attainable for her.

As you can see, by creating some structure around her treatment plan, setting a goal that felt attainable, and tracking the progress, anxiety became more manageable for Jenny. The best part is, although the first twelve months didn't show much improvement, by the end of the second year, she was down to one attack a month. As she continues with this goal-setting process, she reached a point where a whole month recorded no ratings of 10 and no attacks.

That's the journey ahead. It takes courage and requires a commitment. Breaking it down into daily steps really helps, so if Jenny's approach resonates, feel free to borrow it.

The third thing you must do before implementing your daily activities to move toward the objective is to identify the obstacles that might get in the way. There will always be challenges to overcome. If you can identify them and prepare for those obstacles, you will likely handle them without too much strain. For example, if you noticed in Jenny's story, she committed to a 1-minute check-in three times a day and recorded everything on her smartphone. That came from her realization that she hates carrying around journals but doesn't mind voice recording little notes from her phone. She also chose a daily recording system that created minimum resistance for her ensuring she would stay consistent. What obstacles stand in the way of your goal? Is it something technical? Can you find some workarounds?

Another thing I want to note here is that consistency is key. Whatever goal you're working toward, make sure those activities are scheduled so you can create a routine for yourself. For example, if you need to exercise, do it at the same time every day or every week. If you're thought recording like Jenny, do it at the same time each day. Set the alarm to remind you if needed.

WHY MOTIVATION IS NECESSARY

Sometimes even getting out of bed feels impossible. How can you possibly set and achieve goals if taking a shower is a feat of willpower that you seem to be lacking? It's true that mental disorders usually decrease interest in many of the activities we'd otherwise partake in. For example, someone with a social anxiety disorder might set a goal of making seven new friends within twelve months. Still, if she never keeps the commitment of meeting new people, it doesn't matter how perfectly planned her S.M.A.R.T goals are. Lack of motivation can be a huge hindrance to reaching your goals, so if the thought of taking action seems overwhelming, pause for a moment. Breathe deeply and acknowledge that this feels huge for you. Remind yourself that it's not about being perfect or getting it right all the time. Instead, it's about taking small baby steps forward no matter how much you stumble.

Have you ever watched an infant learn how to walk? There is nothing graceful about it, but it is adorable, and we all cheer and commend that baby for each tiny step. It would be best if you parented yourself in this season by acknowledging each small step forward. If the goal is to exercise three times a week at your local gym for forty-five minutes and you only manage thirty minutes a day, that's better than missing your workout. If the squat exercise requires 20 reps and you push all the way to 15 reps, don't think you're a failure. Be grateful and proud that you can do 15 and move on to the program's next exercise. Tomorrow, you'll manage to do 16 reps, and before you know it, 20 reps won't make you feel like passing out. The key to finding that motivation for things that feel impossible is to connect with your why.

Why are you choosing to do this? And why do you think there's so much resistance? Is it because you want to avoid discomfort? Do you doubt yourself? Have you lost hope about healing? The more you can understand the negative driving emotion, the easier it gets to reverse that emotion because you could even give yourself a pep talk. For example, if you feel like you've tried everything, but nothing works, then you could say to yourself, "*I've never really tried it in this order before or using this technique. Besides, it doesn't matter that it hasn't worked the last ten times because I only need it to work once, and I'll be on my way to recovery.*" Sometimes a pep talk and a reminder of why you want to heal is all you need to bring in some motivation.

Meet Dave and Lucy

Dave, a 37-year old manager, had a difficult time at work. He had started his career with plenty of ambition and planned to be one of the greatest in his field. So far, things seemed to be on the right track, but about nine months ago, Dave felt as though he was running out of air while attending a meeting. His heart rate significantly increased; his throat and mouth dried up, and he began to sweat profusely. Although it was a chilly day with clouds covering the sky, he felt as though someone was considerably raising the room's temperature. It felt like sitting in a Sauna while fully clothed. "*Who in their right mind would increase the temperature in the board room, and why was everyone else seemingly calm and normal?*" Dave wondered.

As he tried to pay attention to the presentation, Dave's mind kept wandering and worrying about what he was experiencing and how he could excuse himself from the meeting without raising any concerns. He feared what his colleagues and boss would think. Dave really wanted to protect the seemingly perfect image they had of him. After all, he had spent years working hard on that image, and yet here he sat feeling as though he was about to pass out or, worse yet, die.

After that traumatizing moment, Dave started dreading meetings, especially since he hadn't realized he was experiencing anxiety (more specifically, that he had gotten a panic attack). Each week he would try to come up with some lame excuse so he wouldn't have to go back and face that experience again. Things only got worse after that as he started passing up opportunities to give presentations for fear of messing up or reactivating that same feeling. It wasn't too long before people noticed, and his career started to suffer. He missed a couple of promotions, and suddenly, it dawned on him that he was falling off track.

Dave kept everything to himself for months. He constantly worried over how he felt, which built into a generalized anxiety disorder. His confidence tanked. From the moment he would open his eyes, Dave was stressed and anxious. His wife and friends advised him to "just get over it." They told him he was simply worrying too much, and although they meant well, none of it helped.

On the other hand, Lucy was only 28 when she got convinced that she was very sick. She felt a whole range of strange sensations on a daily basis and couldn't figure out why. Her physician didn't seem to know either. "You're in good health, Lucy. Go home and stop worrying so much" was the usual answer after every hospital visit. Over and over, she heard the same answer. Lucy decided to get a second opinion at the hospital, and still, nothing new was uncovered. A few times, Lucy ended up calling an ambulance because she was convinced her heart was giving up on her. It was at this point that the doctors finally diagnosed her with anxiety. The doctor tending to her said she was too stressed and needed to relax more. Lucy was prescribed anti-depressants, but she refused to take them because she felt it wouldn't help since she wasn't suffering from depression.

The uncertainty of not knowing what was ailing her or how to treat this problem that she knew was there kept her continuously anxious, which only made things worse. Fortunately, Lucy was a fighter, so she decided to go on her own quest and seek answers elsewhere. That's when she turned to the Internet, where she found stories of people who were sick and displaying the same symptoms she had.

Discovering that she wasn't alone and definitely not crazy was a huge relief. But that didn't help her get better. Each week the anxiety was spiking aggressively. Her "illness" was all Lucy could think about, and it started to weigh heavily on her physical health and relationships. Her boyfriend tried to reassure and support her, but nothing was working anymore. The panic attacks were increasing in frequency and intensity. She would have dinner with her boyfriend at times, and out of the blue, she would feel like she's dying, unable to move. Lucy's life got utterly out of hand and more like a circus freak show as everything started crumbling before her. Things she used to enjoy doing, like driving, hiking, and weekend picnics, became impossible.

The consequences of anxiety seriously limited both Dave and Lucy. They tried to cope and even hide it for a while, but eventually, it took a toll on their life. Thanks to the Internet, they connected with me through content and teachings and learned all the book's techniques. Although it was hard to start on the recovery path, one of the ways each of these individuals was able to commit to their treatment path and goals was due to the fact that I encouraged them to reconnect with their "why." For Dave, his big why was healing for his family. As a husband and father, he felt it was paramount that he got his life back on track. Even when it wasn't comfortable, the motivation needed to make an effort was derived from his love and dedication to his family.

On the other hand, Lucy struggled a lot to feel motivated enough to execute her health goals. Some days she struggled to get out of her pajamas. She often had a long list of reasons why not to take action. Then she realized that unless she found a way out of this, she would always be stuck. She desired to start her own business and get married to her boyfriend. None of that would happen unless she completed her treatment and committed to achieving her health goals. As she connected her desires of business and marriage to the daily work of mental healing, motivation grew, and she realized that she could take small steps daily to heal from her anxiety.

Now, there's probably a negative voice in you that might say, "*Sure, but my case is different. I'm probably never going to get better. This won't work for me. It never does. I've already tried so many times.*" Let me remind you that it's okay to have that voice of doubt as it's just trying to protect you. What you must do is compassionately override that suggestion. See it for what it really is - a friendly warning. Your anxiety is actually caused in part by that overly cautious voice of doubt, so once you hear it out, acknowledge that you're not fighting its ideas but merely exploring other possibilities. I mean, what if it does work this time? What if you are not ready to heal? What if your desire to have [fill in the blank] is the big why that was missing from your life. Perhaps now is the time. I believe it's your time. Do you?

HOW TO FIND A THERAPIST BEST SUITED TO YOUR NEEDS & ONE THAT WILL ACTUALLY HELP YOU! (IF YOU NEED ONE, OF COURSE!)

Anxiety disorders can be treated by a wide range of health professionals, including psychologists, psychiatrists, clinical social workers, and psychiatric nurses. But how do you know which is the right one for you? And does everyone need to see a therapist?

First, let me clarify that not everyone needs a therapist to heal from anxiety disorders, but most do. Given that each case is unique and different, I will leave that choice in your capable hands because only you know where you stand and how practical it is for you to do this on your own without professional guidance. On the off chance that you do, in fact, decide to invest in a therapist, here are a few things to consider.

#1: You need to choose a therapist who is right for you. That includes picking the gender, age, and appearance you most resonate with. I'm not saying to look for models or attractive therapists but instead find someone who makes you feel calm, safe, understood, and someone you enjoy being with. After all, this is a relationship that you'll have to commit to. So, if you realize you work best with male or female doctors in general, go for that.

#2: Choose someone who values you as a person and treats you as an equal. There has to be that human connection and empathy going on at all times; otherwise, it won't end well.

#3: Pick a therapist who is relatable, easily accessible, and someone you believe will help you grow and act as the much-needed guide. Finding that "right fit" in this case is very important because this is someone who is qualified medically to walk with you through this challenge and someone who will help you transform from this current you to the new you that you long for. You can think of it as a caterpillar becoming a butterfly. That process isn't going to be easy, but with the right guide, it will take place successfully, and life will never be the same. Does your therapist give you the feeling that he or she is the right person for this quest? If the answer isn't a resounding yes, then you need to keep searching.

THE CONNECTION IS EVERYTHING.

When choosing your therapist, the first and most important thing is to feel a connection between you and them. There has to be some rapport and trust established before you commit to the treatment. A good way for you to feel safe enough to do this is to identify your preferences and match them with your potential therapists. So, don't be afraid to interview as many as will agree. Get to know the person either via a phone call or in-person before making your decision. During the interview, you'll need to have a set of questions to ensure you get the most out of the interaction. Here are a few:

- Are you specialized in treating anxiety disorders?
- How do you approach treating a case like mine?
- How long do you estimate it would take before I can expect to feel better?
- What do you generally do if a patient doesn't feel any better within your typical time frame?
- How can I help in my recovery?
- Why did you choose to become a therapist?
- What credentials and training do you have?
- Are you now, or have you ever been in therapy?
- Do you follow any particular faith (this is especially useful if religion and spirituality matter to you)?

AGREED ON ONE GOAL AND METHOD

Once you've chosen your ideal therapist, the next order of business is to establish a close alliance founded on an agreed-upon vision with corresponding S.M.A.R.T goals for the two of you to collaborate toward. You must be on the same page when it comes to your ultimate objective. A good therapist will desire to agree on how the therapy will progress and how you can work together to meet your goals. It's up to you, however, to show up ready to participate. If you already have your goals identified and know which treatment you prefer, then only work with a therapist who gets that. Alternatively, go for one with whom you feel a connection, and together you can set the right goal and choose the suitable method of treatment.

When it comes to treatment techniques, there are numerous ways to healing mental disorders. Some common types include:

- **Cognitive or cognitive-behavioral therapy:** This is a form of talk therapy that focuses on making connections between thoughts, behavior, and feelings.
- **Client-centered therapy:** This is a non-directive form of talk therapy that emphasizes positive unconditional regard.
- **Existential therapy:** This technique focuses on your free will and self-determination rather than the symptoms.
- **Psychoanalytic or psychodynamic therapy:** This form of treatment focuses on getting in touch with and working through painful feelings in the unconscious mind.
- **Gestalt therapy:** This technique focuses on the "here and now" experiences.

It is essential to consider which treatment resonates with you based on the approach and focus that you want. For example, if you believe there's an unconscious motivation for your anxiety, you might want to see someone who can offer psychodynamic treatment therapy. If you're going to work on your family and not just on your anxiety issues, then perhaps a family-oriented systems therapist might be best. If what you care about is to change thought patterns because you think doing that will change your life, then cognitive therapy treatment will probably be best. If you have no idea what orientation you prefer, discuss it with your therapist either during the interview process or in the first therapy session so you can both agree on the method that feels best for you.

DO CREDENTIALS MATTER?

The formal education that a therapist has is essential, but more integral to your successful treatment is whether you trust him or her. How safe and understood do you feel? Is your therapist continually learning and improving on their knowledge and the latest research regarding your specific disorder? These are the things that will directly impact your treatment and relationship. Just so we are clear, I'm not stating you shouldn't check their license and credentials. Do that for sure but at the same time, listen to your intuition. It shouldn't be enough to settle for a therapist just because they have thirty years of experience and work with celebrities.

MEETING FOR THE FIRST TIME, HERE'S WHAT TO EXPECT

The first meeting with your therapist will be similar to your doctor appointments. It usually involves signing forms, sitting in the waiting room, and waiting for someone to call your name. Of course, if it's a home practice, the experience might be a bit more casual. Some of the forms you'll likely fill include insurance information, medical history (including any current medications), a record release form, a questionnaire about your symptoms, therapist-patient services agreement, and

HIPPA forms. In some cases, you might fill out some of this paper-work before your first session.

What does the first session entail?

The first session is usually different from future visits as this is the first time you sit in-person to know each other and get an idea of how to proceed. Future visits typically follow a more systematic approach focusing on the treatment itself, but a lot of ground has to be covered in this first one. Your therapist will likely ask you what your symptoms are, what brought you to therapy, and other questions regarding your childhood, education, relationships, and life in general.

This is also where you can discuss objectives, treatment options, and the length of your treatment. If there are certain protocols to be employed, he or she will let you know but feel free to raise any concerns and get clarity about how this relationship will work.

Depending on your issue and the chosen method, treatment can last a few sessions, several weeks, or several years. It might be a good idea to agree on a particular timeframe, and you can even ask for the thera-pist's opinion on how long they think it will take before you feel better but understand that there is no set answer. Every patient is different, so at best, you're getting an estimate. But at least it gives you a target and focal point.

If you are paying through insurance, the length of treatment matters even more because some insurance companies only cover a set number of sessions in a given year, so you'll both need to factor in that restriction as you formulate a plan of action.

The last thing I want you to confirm during this first session is to agree upon the method that will be employed to treat your anxiety. Given how diverse therapy can be, you both must agree on an approach based on the options I shared earlier. Your therapist should feel confident and experienced enough to guide you through that specific method. If they lack experience or training in that particular method, I advise you to find someone else because you might not get the best results by forcing it to work.

III

MAKING THE NEW
LIFESTYLE LAST

12

WILL EVERY STEP IN THE GUIDE WORK FOR ME?

Y ou've made it to the last section of the book, where personalizing and implementing your chosen recovery path is the main focus. There's been a lot of information, strategies, and suggestions on approaching and managing your anxiety. We even discussed the possibility of working with a therapist and how to choose a good one.

One thing you need to realize is that you and I respond differently. Therefore, one treatment may work better for you than me. And if you choose to go with a particular treatment and it doesn't yield the results you desire, try adding another. Create combinations that make sense to you because it's okay if the standard rules of recovery fail to apply to your particular case. What matters is that you stick to your healing program and tweak as necessary until the objective is reached. I also want you to remember a couple of important factors as you go through the treatment process.

The first and most important is that your intention must be to work with anxiety, not against it. Steven Hayes, a professor of Clinical Psychology at the University of Nevada in Reno and a man who has experienced his fair share of panic attacks, says we should always be more self-compassionate and accepting during this process. Hayes is the founder of Acceptance Commitment Therapy (ACT), which focuses on acceptance and neutral, non-judgmental observation of negative thoughts. Through this non-resistance, we can more easily come into the present moment and refrain from seeing anxiety as the enemy. The more you make anxiety the enemy, the more your body will wage war essentially against itself. So, whenever the urge arises to make yourself wrong or broken, pause and bring some compassion into the moment. Recognize that an aspect of you is genuinely and chronically afraid, and the right thing to do isn't to deny or push it away, but instead, to bring it close and treat it with some dignity.

You need to remember that you need to spend more time doing things that feel good for you. Do you know what you enjoy? What naturally releases those feel-good hormones? It would help if you got obsessed with this self-discovery because those are the small details that will make your treatment and recovery enjoyable and ultimately successful. I will give you a full outline of how to make a lifestyle shift, but unless the actual activities are fun and feel right for you, they won't be sustainable or produce great results. So, if your thing is yoga or Pilates, that should become your main workout.

DID I CHOOSE THE RIGHT ONE?

Perhaps you might be asking yourself that about many things, including whether this book has been worth the investment. It's normal to need that extra reassurance that you are on the right track and that you've made the right choice. By reading this far into this book, I can already tell you're good at making the right choices because you now have insights that were perhaps missing or unclear before starting this book. And if you've also signed up for a treatment or finally chosen to work with a therapist, that too is what's right for you. If you sometimes start questioning whether it's working during the recovery, consider going through your journal or just thinking back to how things were a few months or years prior.

The recovery period is different for everyone. It might take you several months or years before you feel completely comfortable in your own skin and more aware and in control of your emotions. That doesn't mean things aren't changing in the interim. Each day is a step toward that final objective, and mini-milestones will add up and create a snowball effect. For example, if, thanks to reading this book, you now start your personalized morning and bedtime routine, that's already a sign of recovery. As long as you keep moving forward, you will see progress and results.

If, as a result of reading this book, you feel courageous enough to start facing your fears, feelings and if you feel a sense of hope growing within, then you've already begun making the shift. And the fact that you even got this book, to start with, is a clear example that you have started loving and investing in yourself.

WORKING IT OUT!

It's important to give yourself the necessary time your mind and body need to make the changes permanent. Even if you were to sign up for talk therapy, the shortest sessions for less severe disorders require several weeks and at least eight sessions. That should help you realize that you need to give yourself ample time and that vein fact, the more complex your disorder, the more patience you will need to exercise. Don't put undue pressure on your body to move faster than it can. As long as you track and see tiny bits of improvements, remind yourself that you are healing.

Michelle shares how she learned to develop self-compassion and patience for her healing as it took twelve years to make a significant shift. She was first diagnosed with panic attack disorder which grew into social anxiety, agoraphobia, and severe clinical depression. At her lowest, she was isolated from everyone and started developing suicidal thoughts. All hope was gone, and she just didn't believe there was a way out. Yet twelve years later, she says she barely recognizes herself when she looks in the mirror as she is an entirely different woman. All that unhelpful panic has been eliminated from her life. She loves spending time with friends and family, runs her own business, and enjoys traveling a lot. Michelle now has hobbies, takes holidays, and loves to try new experiences.

A key lesson from Michelle is her realization that panic, anxiety, and depression can be great teachers. They force us to have the courage that we never realized was inside us, and they require us to develop greater compassion, empathy, acceptance, and patience first for ourselves and then for others. But one cannot heal or recover from anxiety unless they are willing to face and feel their own feelings allowing them time to process. That "time" is critical because that's also when healing occurs. According to Michelle, avoidance, and impatience actually keeps the fear cycle alive. That inhibits any progress.

So, one thing you can't afford to do is get impatient or set unrealistic expectations on your healing. Just like Michelle, you are to see your recovery as a quest of self-discovery and self-love. Don't just read this book to tick a box or to satisfy your curiosity. Commit fully without conditions or apprehension, trusting that healing will become inevitable by allowing your body and mind permission to process those painful and dark emotions. You need to develop this self-belief in your powerful ability to restore your quality of life to where you desire it to be so that as you continue on your treatment, it shouldn't be a question of whether or not it will work but instead a declaration that in due time, new success is inevitable.

13

TRULY ACCEPTING YOUR ANXIOUS THOUGHTS & EMOTIONS CAN ACTUALLY HELP YOU DEAL WITH THEM MUCH MORE EFFECTIVELY (TRUE ACCEPTANCE IS DIFFERENT TO WHAT YOU THINK)

A 13th-century poet called Rumi famously compared emotions (joy, depression, etc.) to unexpected visitors. His advice was to let them in laughing. It makes sense, but that's easier said than done. We usually hide, deny or suppress our emotions, especially the negative ones. We're inclined to bury intense feelings like anger and resentment and to suppress or deny loneliness. In a cultural age that's pro-positivity, the pressure to be "happy" and "positive" all the time can be overwhelming to some of us. Most of us try to mask or camouflage what we're feeling, and unfortunately, that only worsens our condition. Think about how many people would be comfortable walking into their office and openly share with colleagues that they are currently battling a mental disorder. Chances are, very few would feel confident enough to share this openly. There's a lot of stigma and shame attached to mental health disorders; therefore, accepting one's condition and those negative emotions becomes challenging. Yet, the invitation is to find a way to practice acceptance and to shift the way we think of anxiety disorder in the first place.

Most people assume acceptance is about making it okay to be sick and powerless. That it's about resigning yourself to a life of dysfunction and constant fear. That's not acceptance; that's defeat!

True acceptance involves being present with the emotion and your current state of discomfort and anxiety without judgment. It's not about denying that you have the problem or even believing that there's no hope for you. Instead, it's about acknowledging that you are still alive, and, despite the current situation, you can and will get better. So, you sit with your feelings and take them for what they are - negative feelings! But as with all emotions and uncomfortable states, they too shall pass, and you will be stronger and better for having lived through that experience.

A few years ago, when Brett Ford (a psychology professor at the University of Toronto) was still a doctoral student at the University of California, Berkeley, she and three fellow Berkeley researchers devised a three-part study in which they were attempting to analyze Acceptance and why it works. Their findings were published in the Journal of Personality and Social Psychology. According to their findings, the magic of acceptance lies in its blunting effect on emotional reactions to stressful events. In other words, accepting dark emotions like rage, anxiety, or hopelessness won't bring you down or amplify the emotional experience. It also won't make you happy (at least not directly), so it leaves you at this neutral place which might be better for your mental health.

THE NEGATIVE EFFECTS OF ANXIETY AND PANIC ATTACKS

Anxiety disorders of any kind are imagination gone evil which triggers chronic fear and stress. Nothing good can arise from such a state. When it comes to the impact living with such a disorder has in your life, the list is long and affects more than just your ability to interact with others. Let's talk about some of the far-reaching effects chronic anxiety and panic attacks can have on you.

Low immune system:

Have you noticed that when you're stressed and anxious, it's easier to "catch something"? That's because when anxiety builds up, your immune system shuts down. After all, the body is under duress. That makes it hard for the body to fight illness and viral infection, so you become very vulnerable to anything in the air.

Weight gain:

Most of us eat more when stressed and anxious, so it's no surprise that our weight will fluctuate as things worsen. There's also the fact that your brain floods your body with hormones of adrenalin and cortisol, which causes most of us to seek out sweet comfort foods like ice cream, cake, and chocolate. However, the rise and subsequent drop in blood sugar levels will lead to a constant craving for salty and sugary foods again. This unending roller coaster can easily lead to weight gain and even obesity if left unchecked.

Gastrointestinal disorders:

The more anxiety builds up, the harder it is to keep your stomach calm. For many of us, the first symptom that something is building is usually butterflies in the stomach. Constant worry and anxiety attacks can create chronic digestion issues and excretory problems (stomach pains, bloating, abdominal cramping, diarrhea, irritable bowel syndrome, vomiting, etc.).

Respiratory issues:

When you get anxious, your breathing becomes short, shallow, and rapid. Your breathing pattern becomes erratic, and you typically experience dizziness, tingling sensations, and at times numbness of the hands and feet. Some people even pass out due to this imbalance between the inhaled oxygen and exhaled carbon dioxide. But even if you don't pass out, this experience of shortness of breath is very uncomfortable. For those with pre-existing respiratory problems like Asthma, the condition might actually worsen. Patients suffering from inflamed airways or chronic obstructive pulmonary disease (COPD) will usually end up in the ER whenever they get a panic attack or anxiety build-up because their system cannot handle that imbalance. So, it becomes even more necessary to keep anxiety and stress in check when one has respiratory problems.

Heart Disease:

Heart palpitations and rapid breathing patterns are common during a panic attack. Unfortunately, as they continue to persist and increase in frequency, this heightened state can cause high blood pressure and coronary problems such as heart disease or heart attack.

Memory loss:

Most people suffering from chronic anxiety report having issues remembering things. They just seem to forget important information, appointments, and so on. That's because generalized anxiety disorder can sometimes impact your short-term memory. If this happens regularly or you realize you're having trouble recalling or keeping up with your hectic schedule, it might be a side effect of the anxiety. Unfortunately, forgetting things might impact your performance at work or school, making you feel more anxious, causing you to fall deeper into that pit of despair.

FACE IT HEAD ON. AVOIDANCE IS NOT THE ANSWER!

There's a culprit that few of us like to discuss because it tends to stir up wrong feelings and agitate the very thing we are trying to cure, but it must be said. Have you ever heard of avoidance coping? Avoidance coping is changing your behavior to avoid thinking about, feeling, or doing something difficult. For example, Have you ever said "No" to an invitation from someone you care about (friend or family member) even though you did want to go to that event/party and show your support? Still, you chickened out because you knew there wouldn't be anyone else there that you would get along with, and the thought of being judged by strangers made you feel anxious? Or perhaps you've had a tense moment at the office with a co-worker. But instead of having that difficult conversation to resolve the issue and voice your frustration, you spend all week going out of your way to avoid them.

You might even ask for a different shift if possible just to avoid seeing or thinking about them. Here's one more that I have been guilty of several times in the past. I used to believe that my relationships were doomed because of my anxiety. And each time I would get into a relationship, it never ended well and didn't last very long. The main reason for my broken relationships always hinged on some unresolved conflict that I didn't want to have. I felt like I just didn't have the stomach to do it, so instead of sticking around to try and work things out, I would often send a text or leave a voice message telling the other person it was over, and I wished them well. More times than not, it would cause my ex to have an emotional outburst which only made me feel worse. At first, I struggled to realize that I was the one with the issue. I couldn't see that I was using avoidance behaviors, so as you read this, you might want to take a moment and reflect on your relationships and how you approach stress. Do you often procrastinate when something feels hard? Do you avoid discussing or facing issues? Make some notes of events or situations where you have used avoidance coping and then realize that something needs to shift.

Avoidance coping is extremely unhealthy for us and, in fact, only exacerbates anxiety. Sure, it feels good to avoid thinking about or doing something at that moment, but the consequences are usually far more stressful. Relying on this as a strategy for stress relief can get out of hand and create more stress. So, what I want you to do is ditch this coping mechanism and instead form healthy habits that build resilience.

What you need to do is to take small steps toward making changes to your behavior. Here's a simple step you can take.

The next time you realize you've just chosen to avoid facing a situation because you're worried about triggering your anxiety, pause and look at your options. You can choose to implement active coping options instead of that harmful avoidance coping strategy. There are two types of active coping options you could choose from: Active-behavioral coping, which addresses the problem directly. Active-cognitive coping which involves changing how you think about the stressor.

So, think about the issue at hand and see if you can reframe your thoughts and identify resources you didn't realize. Perhaps you can recognize hidden benefits in the situation that you didn't notice at first glance. Is it possible to approach the problem from a mental standpoint that doesn't include avoidance? Are there strategies you can actively use that involve doing something different to affect your situation positively?

Going back to the earlier examples that I shared of different scenarios, instead of merely saying "No" to the invitation for fear of being judged by others, let your friend/family member know that you are nervous about attending that party or event. Please share that you would want to support them, but the thought of being left alone in a place where you wouldn't know anyone else causes significant discomfort. Ask the person if they can help make things easier by introducing you to a few of the other attendees or if they could give you some specific practical tasks that would make you feel less alone and more at ease.

When it comes to conflict with a co-worker, rather than avoid them, make a plan to talk with the person and acknowledge that you feel anxious. You could even let them know that this isn't easy for you at the start of the discussion. As part of your plan, please decide on a neutral place to talk that makes you feel at ease and, if needed, enlist the help of another (boss or colleague) to be a mediator, depending on how serious the issue is. I would also suggest including a self-care plan to reward yourself (treat yourself to something nice) after successfully doing this bold thing of facing your fear.

In my case, when I realized that I was guilty of avoidance coping, I started identifying the situations where that occurred. I would immediately turn to my journal to write out what I did and how I would like to do things differently. In some cases, I realized that I still had the chance to take some action and make things right. Then it would be up to me to follow up with some effort. But even when I wasn't able to "fix" my error, I still wrote down my emotions and how I would do things differently. This gave me that sense of relief and the ability to face my fears, albeit on paper. So instead of escaping things, I gradually got better and faced them head-on.

TEARS OF HOPE

In 1998 a movement known as positive psychology (PP) was launched, and it quickly gained momentum in contemporary psychology. As with everything else, there's been a maturity of sorts as people seek out something more holistic that doesn't just focus on being positive all the time. That's where the second wave of positive psychology comes into play as it promises to be more balanced and inclusive. In theory, PP 2.0 recognizes that it is scientifically and experientially indefensible to only focus on positive emotions, positive traits, and positive institutions. This is a very good thing for us, you know why? Because for people dealing with mental disorders, this idea of being positive all the time only makes things worse. We can't just switch off anxiety, and we certainly can't feel happy when we're not. So, where does that leave us?

This second wave aims to give us an answer. Essentially it makes it okay for us to acknowledge and even embrace our dark and undesirable feelings. So instead of sitting on the couch loathing yourself for having dark intrusive thoughts that make you want to crawl into a hole in the ground, PP 2.0 says it's okay. Just sit with your dark, uncomfortable emotions and cry if you must but remind yourself that it's okay. You are okay. Nothing is wrong with you for having negative emotions. Observe how your mind will just pick up negative emotions and serve them to you on a platter. Realize that while you may not have access to happy utopia-like thoughts and emotions, it's still on the menu, and eventually, you might catch a glimpse of that too. But for now, you'll just accept yourself as you are and feel proud for noticing and becoming aware of these disturbing emotions. Think back to the setting that might have landed you in this undesirable place. Is it lack of sleep? Were you thinking about a setback or troubling experience that happened? Is it too much stress? Are you struggling in some way? Usually, there's a trigger that causes this negative state to kick into high gear. The more you can identify those triggers, the better. But even if you can't recall what triggered you, the fact that you're here sitting with your negativity and feeling uncomfortable is good enough to start practicing PP 2.0. How does one do this?

How to handle negative emotions without resisting them:

Remember, what you resist persists. We want you to have a healthy way of facing and processing the negative emotions and intrusive thoughts that come. To do that, we're going to employ a mnemonic technique gaining worldwide popularity for its effectiveness.

A researcher named Ceri Sims published the mnemonic "TEARS HOPE" in a journal titled "Second Wave Positive Psychology Coaching with Difficult Emotions" that you can implement anytime negative emotions show up. Here's how this method works.

T (Teach and Learn): This is about enhancing your self-awareness and knowledge of your mind-body connection. The purpose is to learn how your body and mind respond to stress and why you have panic attacks. There's always a driving reason behind it, and it's essential to understand it.

E (Express and enable sensory and embodied experiences): Be curious and remain conscious of all that your body is experiencing. Notice all sensations and be okay with whatever is showing up without judgment or resistance. *For example, when my heart rate increases and my stomach tightens up in knots, I simply deepen my breath, stop whatever I'm doing, and repeat to myself that it's okay. Whatever is coming, I will sit my body and just ride the wave. It creates great comfort for my brain.*

A (Accept and befriend): The intention here is to accept whatever emotions or sensations you're having—practice self-compassion and tolerance for that frustration and discomfort.

R (Re-appraise and reframe): This is where you use your preferred method of therapeutic technique to help you see the broad perspective of things. You want to reframe your thoughts and shift your view about the events that are taking place. Cognitive-behavioral approaches can be great for this step.

S (Social support): This is where you engage in a practice that will enable you to find calmness and practice loving kindness. You could do a loving-kindness meditation which will expand your sense of connectedness with yourself and others.

H (Hedonic well-being or Happiness): This is where you shift your focus to happy memories, success stories, and all the positive aspects of your life. Why? Because research shows, it's highly beneficial to keep a 3:1 ratio of positive vs. negative emotions. Practically speaking, you would need to increase the amount of time you spend authentically feeling good. So, when you do catch that good feeling, make sure you ride it as long as possible.

O (Observe): This is where you practice non-judgment in your life. Again, meditation and other mindfulness practices can be integrated here.

P (Physiology): This is where you integrate breathing techniques, relaxation, and self-care exercises.

E (Eudaimonia): This is an ancient Greek term that can be loosely translated to mean human flourishing and happiness. In this context, its purpose is to encourage you to have goals that you're moving toward. Goals that thrill and excite you and enable you to lead a more authentic life that fulfills you.

Turn the Negative to Positive (I was able to do it, now it's your turn):

Anxiety by itself is neither good nor bad, in my opinion. It's mainly the relationship we have with it that determines how it impacts our lifestyles. To prove this, I want to share a story from a fellow community member named Rosie.

As a child, Rosie was very outgoing. She studied ballet and tap dance, joined the school chorus, and even performed in school plays. The spotlight was something Rosie enjoyed, and it suited her. Other kids would complain of pre-show jitters whenever they were getting ready for a big performance, and Rosie never understood why. Feeling nervous was foreign to her. One day, something changed. Suddenly, like the flip of a switch, Rosie found herself feeling tense, scared, and afraid to speak in front of her classmates (there were only 20 kids in the room). What happened? She experienced a key triggering event that activated her anxiety. In February 2001, a classmate vomited all over her while they were riding the school bus. Like any other child, she was grossed out! Although she felt humiliated and unable to control the incident, she didn't think much of it until the next day when she felt frightened to get on the bus or even go to school. The thought of seeing her friend's face after that event made her completely nauseous, and for the next three days, she never left home. Her parents tried to be understanding and let her take some time to process her emotions. She kept insisting that going to school would make her fall ill, so they let her have it easy until finally, they forced her to go back. Once she returned, things weren't normal anymore. She began to see her school guidance counselor to avoid any situation that made her nervous. These visits became so frequent that her parents were alerted, and Rosie was advised to start seeing the school psychologist. Her parents did their best to support and encourage her. Each visit brought no improvement despite her willingness to show up, so the doctor suggested medication. The parents stubbornly refused as they were concerned this would only lead to long-term addiction and further harm to their little girl.

Daily life continued to prove challenging for Rosie. Not long after, she dropped all her extra-curriculum activities and became invisible during class activities. Her engagement level both at home and school dropped significantly. At this point, the parents decided to hire a therapist to help keep the anxiety at bay. The treatment suggested by the therapist seemed to help Rosie maintain her classes, but her social life never recovered. Rosie became a recluse and spent most of her late teenage years grappling with bouts of depression and moving from one therapist to the next. By the time she was in her twenties, her parents had invested a fortune in her well-being and finally found a therapist who was able to teach Rosie some healthy coping mechanisms including, nighttime rituals that included meditation, daily journal, and thought tracking and practicing non-judgment. Rosie says her mother has been a strong influence in her recovery because she never gave up hope and always encouraged her.

Over the years, her anxiety evolved and included obsessive-compulsive behavior, agoraphobia, social anxiety, and bouts of depression. Rosie got to a point where she would only leave the house to go to school and the hospital. The idea of flying, riding buses, or socializing devastated her. Even as a college graduate, she spent each day agonizing over things that normal girls would scoff at and spent all her free time locked up in her room or crying in her mother's lap. Eventually, she did make an effort to conquer her fears and anxiety, and once she found my materials and joined our supportive community, she's been able to reclaim her life. The last posting, she did was actually during her second cross-Atlantic journey, which didn't require any medication (although she still likes to carry some Xanax just in case). It has been 14 years since that trigger moment, and while Rosie's journey hasn't been a bed of roses, she is living proof that it is possible to take back control of your life. It took several therapists, lots of experimentation, and effort on her part, not to mention family support. And she feels confident that the next 14 years will be full of adventure and freedom.

I feel the same way, and my relationship with anxiety has changed tremendously. I cannot say that I will never have another panic attack, but I can assure you, I will handle whatever comes. I have made peace with the fact that the present moment and my emotions are all I can ultimately control. So, I leave the future where it is and trust that I have enough tools, healing coping strategies, and a solid belief in myself to handle anything, including another anxiety attack. Thus far, my streak of anxiety-free days continues to reign, and I savor every minute of it!

WOULD YOU LIKE A NEW WAY OF LOOKING AT ANXIETY, SO YOU COME OUT FEELING EMPOWERED?

Consider viewing it as a protective mechanism. See it as a message from your brain and body. Notice when it shows up and try to understand the signals and messages being sent. Stress and fear, which often trigger anxiety, are both protection mechanisms. Like a fight or flight instinct, anxiety might be your body letting you know that you're in the proximity of danger. Whether that danger is emotional or physical, real or imagined, the signals are accurate, and you should never ignore or judge them as bad. The way you choose to view your anxiety will determine how quickly you can heal. See it as a villain, and you're basically at war with your own body. Instead of making it the bad guy, see if you can "team-up" to resolve the underlying and real problem.

14

WHAT' SPIRITUAL GREATS' LIKE THE BUDDHA CAN TEACH YOU ABOUT HEALING YOUR ANXIETY (WITHOUT HAVING TO BE RELIGIOUS OR SPIRITUAL, IF YOU DON'T WANT TO BE!)

For a long time, I thought mental illness was something experienced by those who were broken somehow. Of course, that tells you a lot about how I viewed myself. Through personal education and increasing my awareness of faith, religion, and spirituality, I've come to realize that many people learn to live with and even overcome mental health disorders. Sometimes, those people are highly respected religious and spiritual leaders. That's why I include this as one of the last chapters in the book. Buddhism is in many ways connected to almost any spiritual or religious practice I can think of, which makes it ideal whether you want to add it to an existing tradition or as a standalone practice.

Perhaps you've never considered spirituality or religion to be of value. Maybe you gave it up because you felt it wrong to claim to be a person of faith, all the while battling with a mental illness. I met a woman who told me she felt so sinful about her depression diagnosis and figured she should as well quit going to church every week because God doesn't like sinners.

I don't know where you stand when it comes to faith, church, religion, or even spirituality, and quite frankly, it doesn't matter. What does matter is that you develop a personal belief in yourself and your ability to heal. How you reach there will be unique to you. But I hope you can pick a few inspiring and insightful lessons from reading about how global figures like the Buddha and lesser-known individuals like Jude Demers have found peace through Buddhism.

Who is Jude Demers? She's a practicing Buddhist who lives with mental illness. Demers says, "Buddhism is known as the science of the mind." I like that definition because it puts us squarely in the arena of personal discovery. By practicing Buddhism not as a religion but as a lifestyle, you become the "scientist" of your own mind and life, experimenting to see what works for you. As you develop and train your mind, inner peace becomes a reality. That's what we're here to discover - how to find peace. We know that as your mind finds peace, your anxiety and fears will dissolve into nothingness. So, where does one begin?

FINDING YOUR PEACE WITHIN

Peace can be defined in a myriad of ways, depending on your source. I am going to broadly define it as the state you experience when what you say, think, feel, and do are in alignment. That can only happen when you become true to yourself and start leading an authentic life. Most people are shocked when I tell them to stop looking for a magic switch that will take away all discomfort, negative feelings, unpleasant situations, and stress in life. Peace will not be yours because you live in a perfect world; it can only be yours when you become a master of your mind.

The more you can align with your values and live in accordance with that, the easier it will be to start making this shift. Peace is dynamic, and it requires courage if you want to live peacefully on a daily, weekly, and monthly basis.

The main form of mental training is meditation. Scientific studies show that meditation can reduce anxiety when practiced over time as you will learn to see negative thoughts and emotions from a different perspective. Instead of letting thoughts nag and steal your peace, you can learn to recognize and release unproductive thoughts. By the way, you don't have to sit in a lotus position for hours each day to practice meditation. Deep breathing, yoga, and chanting are all powerful ways of practicing meditation and mindfulness. Whichever method works to get you to that state of nirvana (the mental state of peace and happiness) is what you should consider implementing.

Here's the thing. You've spent a significant amount of time living in the reality of negative thinking and feeling. The turbulence you experience is real. Practicing meditation in Buddhism isn't about denying that instead of transcending from that viewpoint to a new and more liberating one. If you're more of a religious person, you can also use meditation as a form of prayer to receive the same benefits.

From a Buddhist perspective, the root cause of all suffering is that we don't take enough time through prayer and meditation to come to know ourselves, i.e., our true nature and our enlightened "Buddha" mind. Let's see if we can help you take a step in the right direction by the end of this chapter.

TRANSCENDING FEAR BY UNCOVERING THE SOURCE

One of the great teachings one can learn from Buddhism is that our suffering and fears generally stem from our impermanence and the impermanence of all things. Think about it for a moment. There's so much fear around death, losing our loved ones, losing our precious material possessions, and so on. We're afraid to lose our job or a stock market trade or an ongoing war, and most of all, we're so scared that we will fail. That fear of failure stems from a belief of being unworthy and not good enough. Despite the fears that torment your mind, uncovering the source is the fastest way to tame that voice of anxiety.

You can discover its source through the path of self-inquiry (introspection) or the practice of looking within, which is often part of Buddhism. For instance, suppose fear of death is at the source of your anxiety. Having enough courage to look at it boldly, you'd soon realize that there's another healthier way of thinking about death. You could ask yourself the question, "If everything dies and changes, then what is really true? Is there something behind the appearances? Is there something I can depend on that does survive death?"

If you could spend time in contemplation of these types of questions, you'd notice a shift in the way you view everything. Letting go of this fear will seem more natural because you will see avoidance of the natural cycle of life is actually working against your very nature. As you discover the truth about this particular fear, healing would occur. In essence, what we need to do to activate healing in our minds is to observe with mindfulness, be fully present with whatever is there, and accept. That is where transformation takes place.

THE DIALOGUE IN YOUR HEAD DOES NOT DEFINE YOU

Have you noticed there's ongoing chatter 24/7 in your mind? If you have, what tone does it possess? Is it empowering or disempowering? I remember when I first became aware of my inner dialogue. It was frightening to me that all that negative self-talk was carrying on without my conscious knowledge.

I would walk into a restaurant or coffee shop and find the darkest, most secluded spot, walk to my seat all the while, noticing the people who were staring at me like I was some lost weirdo. All that harsh judgment that seemingly sat on the faces of strangers was actually brewed within my mind first through my inner dialogue. The story I was telling myself was what my ego believed. *I'm a failure at everything. People think I'm stupid and weird. I'm stuck with this sickness. I will never be successful or find love.* On and on it went. What did I do? Nothing, because I didn't have enough awareness to realize that it was just a story. Many of us have lived the "story" of being mentally ill for so long; we don't even know it's a made-up story. You could just as easily start telling the story of "*I am healthy and healed*," but your ego would just scoff and say you're ridiculous because it's so accustomed to telling the story of sickness. I bet throughout this book you've had many moments where that inner dialogue took over and discouraged you or said things like, "*this can't work for you; you already tried these strategies before. What a waste of money buying this book!*"

That inner dialogue has been the blueprint that your ego lives by, and unless you do something to change that story, no amount of medication, talk therapy, or lifestyle changes will give you the life of your dreams. Automatic inner dialogue is a real thing, and it's time you pay attention to what you're telling yourself. A friend of mine told me how he recently caught himself replaying a scene in his mind of getting rejected at a job interview for something he felt so qualified for. There was a little voice in the back of his head saying, "*you'll never get the job; you're not skilled enough.*" That discouraging process caused him so much anxiety and mental exhaustion. He would have triggered a full-blown panic attack if he hadn't been quick enough to catch his inner speech.

Sometimes the inner dialogue isn't even directed at you. It might be focused on judging other people, commenting on what's going on, arguing internally with you know or don't know, and so much more. These activities can quickly become triggers for your anxiety and panic attacks.

Buddhism has teachings on how to deal with this inner dialogue. It involves coming to a place of self-observation to perceive with awareness and clarity these conversations and realize that we are not our thoughts. The true self (who you really are) is not the ego or the mind where this inner dialogue is taking place. Through increased self-awareness, you can learn to detach from all the mind's mental processes and activities and simply observe.

How to start turning your inner conversation into more constructive thoughts:

- Become aware of the conversation you're having and calmly try to observe (like an investigator or a director of a movie) the activity in your mind.
- Strive to keep your attention on what's going on inside your head. You might keep getting distracted but do your best to come back to observing until you can reach that point of detachment (between you and your mental activity and thoughts).
- Find that damaging or futile conversation, stop it, and switch it to something more useful and meaningful. Think of it like switching from one radio station to another. Replace the subject and the words with something more pleasant.

YOU AND I ARE CONNECTED; YOU ARE NOT ALONE

In spirituality, we understand that much of our suffering is enhanced by a sense of separation and being alone. So, one of the first steps to healing that self of loneliness is to reconnect oneself with life and others. Surprisingly, this can also alleviate the tension and nervousness we usually feel, especially if we are convinced that no one "gets us" or loves us. You need to realize that you are not alone. All of us have experienced that debilitating pain of living with anxiety, and though it manifests differently for each of us, we all share that pain. And those of us who have found a way to overcome and rebuild our lives are still connected to you and can be there for you if you will allow it. The same is true with your loved ones. If you can find a way to connect with those you care about deeply, whether they are alive or not, you can learn to tap into the same power taught by Buddha and all the other great spiritual teachers. How do you do this? You can sit in meditation regularly and connect yourself to the people you love and those across the world like me who support and cheer for your well-being. Focus on your breath and bring that mindfulness into the moment. Imagine yourself surrounded by people who love you. Feel yourself touching the shoulder of a loved one next to you and express your love, gratitude, and compassion. Breathe in the knowing that you are not alone, for we are all in this together. As you heal and bring your mind to a state of oneness, we all become better human beings, and the world becomes a healthier, brighter place.

WHY WOULD YOU WANT TO TAKE A MORE SPIRITUAL APPROACH?

Although you don't "have to" become spiritual or religious to heal from anxiety, many who have chosen to follow this path claim it was the best decision ever made (myself included). Why?

First and foremost, it moves one from a self-centeredness approach and that feeling of being alone into a state of connectedness. If you think about it, anxiety is rooted in fear and thoughts such as *"I'm not good enough. What will happen to me? What do people think of me? What's wrong with me?"* etc.

Notice that all these thoughts are very focused on ME. It's an ego-centered approach to living which hinges on external circumstances going right. When they don't, which is at least 50% of the time, anxiety kicks in. The problem with this way of being is that one can never get enough external validation. Also, life is full of both positive and adverse conditions. So, this approach can only keep recreating cause for hopelessness, fear, and anxiety.

When we turn our lives around and seek out spiritual solutions, we shift our focus to "something larger than ourselves." Some might call it God if they are religious. Others may settle for Higher Purpose, Higher Power, or Source. When the focus is taken away from the ego, the perspective changes. For example, we realize that death happens to all of us, and it happens every second of every minute. In fact, by the time I finish typing this sentence, at least two people have passed away somewhere in this world. We also shift from trying to protect and satiate the ego and start asking questions such as *"what is my purpose? Whom can I serve today? What can I do for another to make them feel that they are not alone? What is the right thing for me to think and do at this moment? What is this anxiety teaching me about myself?"*

By connecting to something larger than yourself, you are relieved from the bondage of the ego-self and all the self-obsessed fears and neuroses that typically accompany ego thoughts. Spiritual practices like meditation and prayer can help you recognize and detach from the emotional reactions that usually trigger panic. In essence, you learn how to connect to the part of yourself that is always calm, peaceful, and happy. You also learn to love yourself just as you are, including the dark aspects of your personality. And when it comes to your anxiety disorder, let's just say it's easier to change your viewpoint and emotions around having it in the first place. That health issue becomes an opportunity for growth and expansion instead of a hindrance. You begin to believe that nothing is going wrong, and you are moving through life precisely as your soul designed it to be so you can express and discover more of who you really are. Instead of succumbing to the torture of living with anxiety, you begin to rise stronger, better, wiser, and more compassionate than ever because you see your life through a different lens for the first time in your life. I am not advocating for any particular religion or spiritual approach. Whatever works for you is fine as long as you feel deep within that something larger than yourself is calling you into a new experience. And if spirituality is your path, follow it wholeheartedly and trust that your purpose will lead the way.

15

THE 1 LIFE-CHANGING PIECE OF ADVICE TO HELP MAKE YOUR NEW ANXIETY-FREE LIFESTYLE STICK, AND WHAT TO DO WHEN THE ANXIETY COMES BACK

The recovery path will come with challenges. Even after treatment is done and you find yourself experiencing fewer panic attacks and more joy-filled productive days, there's no guarantee you will never have another anxiety breakdown again. That might sound grim, but it is, in fact, good news for you because what that implies is that you don't need to concern yourself with never having anxiety again! Instead, you need to focus on taking each day at a time, doing the best you can to be present and in control of your emotions. Above all else, you need to set yourself up for success by developing the right habits and cultivating the right mindset.

If there's one bulletproof way to enjoy an anxiety-free lifestyle, it must be the cultivation of the right mindset. Your frame of mind will determine how healthy, happy, productive, and fulfilled you become. That includes training your mind to accept and embrace all emotions, including the negative ones without attachment. It's also about decluttering your inner and outer world. Notice your living space and working space. How serene and organized is it? Notice your internal dialogue and mental space. How chaotic and cluttered are things? Are you exposing yourself to negative news, gossip, and unhelpful conversations or feeding it rich, healthy, prosperous information? It's vital to keep analyzing your inner and outer environment so you can clean up and declutter whatever clogs that sense of serenity. In her book, The Life-Changing Magic of Tidying Up, by Marie Kondo tells us to "Focus on the things you want to keep, not on the things you want to get rid of." So, if you can identify what you want to keep doing and start getting rid of everything else that doesn't support or serve a purpose in your life, you'll feel a tremendous shift in your emotional, mental, and physical health.

THAT ONE LIFE-CHANGING ADVICE TO STICKING TO YOUR NEW LIFESTYLE

If there's one piece of advice I'd like you to carry for the rest of your life, it's this. It's okay to have a setback because setbacks don't make you a failure. There's nothing wrong with you if anxiety strikes a year or so after you've healed your mental disorder. The only time failure occurs is when you give up on taking care of your mental health. Most people assume they should only and always go forward in their healing process. But life is never that black and white. Sometimes you might take two steps forward and one step back. That "setback" is still progress in my eyes and should never be seen as a negative.

Recognize that leftover automatic negative thoughts (ANTs) may be playing a mind game with you, so you need to stop them as soon as you catch yourself and then calmly and gently redirect your focus. If you have therapy handouts of processes that have been helping you throughout this process, now would be the best time to implement some of those exercises to ground yourself in the present moment. You could even say something as simple as "Wait! I'm not going to give in to my negative thoughts and emotions. I've been so long without an incident, and I know my body is healing. These thoughts are just irrational lies that make things seem worse than they are. I know I will be okay no matter what, and it's okay if right now I don't feel so good. I will still be okay. I choose not to go down the pigpen. I'm tired of wallowing in the mud. Been there, done that. I don't need to torture myself like that. Instead, I will "make" myself sit here, embrace myself, and just breathe." Of course, this is easier said than done. Sometimes you might need a more impactful exercise to create that shift, so just be present and utilize one of the tools in your distress kit.

A SETBACK DOES NOT SET US BACK, BUT WHY DO WE HAVE IT?

As you go through your recovery, you will have a real glimpse of the fact that the old you is still there, especially when those leftover automatic negative thoughts kick in. And you'll also become reacquainted with the real you who got buried underneath all your symptoms. You will have days of total clarity, sharp thinking, and freedom, and that sense of joy and purpose that you've always wanted will fill you up. One day, you might wake up and feel like you're back to square one. On those days, everything will feel like a struggle, and you might feel like you're failing, and healing isn't really happening. When that happens, you need to remember that your mind and body go through cycles, and some seasons will be more challenging than others. When your mind starts to feel noisy, detached, and nervous, stay open to whatever is showing up. Don't make it wrong or try to manipulate the moment because setbacks happen even to the best of us. I am convinced that setbacks happen when real healing is taking place.

As your mind and body readjusts and frees up old energies, things will happen. You need to understand that there is no quick fix or shortcut for healing, and everyone takes however much time they need for a full recovery. The more you resist, fight, and interfere with the natural healing process, the harder it will be to transform your health and life.

Consider what happens when someone does a detox or goes into a physical fast. At first, everything feels okay, but you reach a point where it feels awful, and your body might even feel sick and worse than before. This seeming setback is actually the turning point. Usually, people will give up because it just gets too hard. But the few who stick with it and ride that discomfort always find themselves on the other side, ultimately victorious. Just as the body needs to get rid of the toxins before it can be cleansed and energized, so too will your mind. The best you can do is ride out these discomforts and seeming setbacks trusting that once that storm passes, you'll be stronger, better, and well on your way to that new lifestyle.

So, there's no need to worry about why setbacks happen or to feel bad when you're not mentally at your best. What matters is that you are accepting and understanding of your healing process. The ups and downs of recovery from anxiety are the natural processes of healing. It won't just be smooth sailing, and that is okay.

Ben, who I helped recover from panic attacks, shared this message based on his own experience with setbacks which might give you the comfort and perspective needed.

"Setbacks have always been an interesting experience for me. Hopefully, I'm not the only one who feels that way. My setbacks felt like they destroyed everything I had been fighting for. I'd be coming out of the pit, and then I'll wake up one morning only to be met with that profound sense of dread, despair, and loss. Good times can sometimes feel like a hoax, and that little evil voice often whispers that peace and happiness cannot be real. That the only reality was the nightmare of anxiety and panic attacks and all the symptoms that go along with it. When you have those episodes, it's easy to believe that nothing will ever get better. At a fundamental level, that was one of my biggest hurdles. Changing that belief that I am broken, and there's no hope for me has been a massive task. I think experts call it an automatic negative reaction. Willfully, I had very little power over just changing that belief. I would argue with it, try to read the same things that once gave me hope, only to fall flat on my face. At one point, my despair was so bad I literally felt like there was nothing more to do but die. But it was at that moment that I realized I had two choices. I could wallow in my despair and wait to die, or I could get up and take a step forward, fully accepting of the fact that I am having a rough patch, but my emotions are not the totality of my life. I believe that was my point of redemption. In recognizing the futility of fighting with my fears, symptoms, and thoughts, I started to live my life wholeheartedly regardless of my state. Then something crazy started happening. The dark clouds seemed to dissipate, and that awful feeling of failure lost its grip on me. How is this happening? I asked myself. Despite all those negative emotions, I started feeling that I wasn't broken. I felt that in time, this storm would pass. And indeed, it passed and has continued to do so ever since. It's almost like when I stopped fighting and resisting setbacks, that surrender allowed peace to enter my mind and body. And almost every time I had a setback, once I came out of it, it was like a little piece of me was restored back."

MOVING FORWARD WITH SETBACKS!

The length of your setback should never be an issue. What matters is that you have the right attitude and the willingness to accept, process, and keep moving forward, as Ben shared. Increase your awareness and understanding of what's happening when you have a setback so you can allow yourself to have a great life at last. If you would like some tips on how to handle those challenging moments in a healthy way, here are a few things to practice. Know that sometimes, none of these will work, and that's okay.

Find all your achievements no matter how small and celebrate:

Since most of us feel helpless and drained of the previously gained knowledge and progress, a good exercise is to remind yourself of how far you've come. There has been evidence of success (no matter how small), and it's important to recall or read from your journal all the days where things felt great. Did you manage to work out and hit all your weekly goals? Great. Celebrate that old win again. Show yourself all the times you've overcome a challenge.

Get back to basics:

Don't feel ashamed of going back to the basic techniques and principles that first got you moving if you have handouts from your therapy sessions or books that were helpful, re-read those.

Deep breathing techniques and mindfulness practices:

Go back to practicing breathing and relaxation techniques. Remember the deep breathing exercises, meditation, and grounding exercises that you learned earlier in the book? Implement those religiously.

Create your personalized flashcards:

It's hard to remember helpful affirmations, statements, or tips when in the midst of a setback. Consider creating some flashcards that you can pull out when you're about to fall into despair. You could write statements such as:

I have a setback which is why I feel like this, but it's okay. I am still OK.

I will feel better again. I've recovered before, and I will do it again.

Setbacks are a normal part of recovery.

CONCLUSION

Congratulations on making it to the end of this book. It's been a wild, emotionally challenging ride. Your commitment shall be greatly rewarded if you follow up and implement everything you've learned. Anxiety is like wearing dark-colored sunglasses. Everything seems gloomy no matter what you're looking at. I know going through this book has had its fair share of challenges, and so will completing your treatment. But once you find yourself on the other side of anxiety, those dark glasses will vanish, and you will finally enjoy the freedom and fulfillment you've been dreaming of.

Let's remind ourselves once more that negative thoughts and distorted thinking won't vanish forever. Along this journey, you will still find yourself thinking and feeling negatively toward yourself and others. When that happens, observe without judgment and allow them to drift on by. Negative thinking and beliefs are never easy to change and will require time. Positive affirmations are great, but they may not always work, so what you need is to develop the right awareness and practice mindfulness as a way of life. Be proactive and take steps on your own whether you work with a therapist or not. By the way, as we discussed earlier, getting professional help doesn't make you weak or crazy. If you need some support, consider hiring a therapist that feels like the right fit. Working with a therapist can provide you with the objectivity, accountability, and guidance most necessary in the healing process. It can be a way for you to create a "safe space" for you to explore, share, discuss, and examine the cause of your anxiety. It can also be the best solution to have a professional supporting you as you learn life skills for overcoming it.

In our volatile economy and social media-addicted society, mental health issues are a real challenge for many young adults, so don't feel there's something wrong with you. Treatment of emotional problems is critical for our generation if we wish to enjoy modern civilization and maintain a sense of peace and happiness.

The bottom line is, peace and happiness matter to us, and we should do everything we can to retrain our minds the same way we emphasize training our physical bodies. Some people can do it on their own at home with a YouTube video, while others require a gym membership with a personal trainer to make it work. There is no right or wrong. What matters is that it gets you the results you want. When it comes to mental health, you can choose to embark on this quest by yourself and follow the recommendations outlined in this book, or you can combine these ideas with the support of a community/ therapist, depending on what feels best. Here's what I know for sure. You cannot permanently heal and transform your life if all you're looking for are shortcuts or quick fixes. The mind cannot be cheated or short-changed into transformation. You will need to step up and take responsibility. Learn to face your fears, and accept your wild, unruly, and sometimes dark emotions. Invest in anything and everyone who helps you expand your self-awareness because everything begins and ends with you. The quality of life you will have as you take the next steps are not dependent on the economy, how bad your anxiety gets, or where you live. Your quality of life depends on you and the choices you make daily. So, my invitation is for you to start making life-giving choices. Decide that you will invest some time experimenting with new morning and nighttime rituals. Choose to adjust your current nutrition, workout habits, and sleep habits. Integrate mindfulness as a way of life. Invest in more books, teachers, events, or even group therapy sessions where you can have access to like-minded, inspiring people. Peace and happiness have never been missing in your life. You just need to learn ways of eliminating or avoiding the things that cause you to block out these beautiful states.

Most people will pick up this book with the perspective that anxiety is terrible, and they are flawed and broken. I hope that by now, you've started to see things differently. That you've realized anxiety, panic, or any other disorder cannot rule your life unless you hand over your mind and let it be on the driver's seat. I also hope that you realize that no matter how bad things have been, they can change for the better. Today can be the start of your new life. You can find peace and happiness now even as you recover and heal from anxiety. Make-believe that your new life is real and that it's time for you to have a better quality of life, and that is precisely what you will get.

Thank you for reading my story, the story of others just like us who have walked the same path and proven that freedom is possible. And last but not least, thank you for still believing in yourself. Go forth and heal.

RESOURCES PAGE

Oakley, A. (2016, August 24). Your Natural State Of Being. Retrieved February 27, 2021, from https://www.innerpeacenow.com/inner-peace-blog/natural-state-of-being

Three common misconceptions about anxiety. (n.d.). Retrieved February 27, 2021, from https://www.beyondblue.org.au/personal-best/pillar/in-focus/three-common-misconceptions-about-anxiety

Anxiety disorders - Symptoms and causes. (2018, May 4). Retrieved February 27, 2021, from https://www.mayoclinic.org/diseases-conditions/anxiety/symptoms-causes/syc-20350961

Three common myths about anxiety. (2018, August 10). Retrieved February 27, 2021, from https://www.trainingjournal.com/articles/features/three-common-myths-about-anxiety

Common Misconceptions About Anxiety Disorders. (2020, November 5). Retrieved February 27, 2021, from https://www. banyanmentalhealth.com/2018/08/02/common-misconceptions-about-anxiety-disorders/

Stöppler, M. C. (2007, January 1). Panic Attack Symptoms. Retrieved February 27, 2021, from https://www.webmd.com/anxiety-panic/guide/panic-attack-symptoms

NIMH » Social Anxiety Disorder: More Than Just Shyness. (2021, March 3). Retrieved February 27, 2021, from https://www.nimh.nih.gov/health/publications/social-anxiety-disorder-more-than-just-shyness/index.shtml

Harvard Health Publishing. (2020b, October 13). Yoga for anxiety and depression. Retrieved February 27, 2021, from https://www.health.harvard.edu/mind-and-mood/yoga-for-anxiety-and-depression#:%7E:text=By%20reducing%20perceived%20stress%20and,blood%20-pressure%2C%20and%20easing%20respiration.

High-Intensity Exercise Best Way To Reduce Anxiety, University Of Missouri Study Finds. (n.d.). Retrieved February 27, 2021, from https://www.sciencedaily.com/releases/2003/07/030715091511.htm

Bonfil, A. (2020, August 26). Mindfulness from a DBT Perspective. Retrieved February 27, 2021, from https://cogbtherapy.com/cbt-blog/mindfulness-in-dbt

Khoramnia, S. (n.d.). The effectiveness of acceptance and commitment therapy for social anxiety disorder: a randomized clinical trial.

Retrieved February 27, 2021, from http://www.scielo.br/scielo.php?script=sci_arttext&pid=S2237-60892020000100030

Gavlick, K. (2020, March 15). Breathe In, Breathe Out: Simple Breathwork Meditation For Beginners. Retrieved February 27, 2021, from https://www.organicauthority.com/energetic-health/breathe-in-breathe-out-simple-breathwork-meditation-for-beginners

Connection Between Mental and Physical Health. (n.d.). Retrieved February 27, 2021, from https://ontario.cmha.ca/documents/connection-between-mental-and-physical-health/

Exercise for Stress and Anxiety | Anxiety and Depression Association of America, ADAA. (n.d.). Retrieved February 27, 2021, from https://adaa.org/living-with-anxiety/managing-anxiety/exercise-stress-and-anxiety

How to Design the Ideal Bedroom for Sleep. (2020, October 23). Retrieved February 27, 2021, from https://www.sleepfoundation.org/bedroom-environment/how-to-design-the-ideal-bedroom-for-sleep

rockland-editor. (2016, July 26). How to Develop Coping Skills for Anger, Anxiety, and Depression. Retrieved February 27, 2021, from http://www.rocklandhelp.org/how-to-develop-coping-skills-for-anger-anxiety-and-depression/

Understanding Anxiety Disorders. (2017, September 8). Retrieved February 27, 2021, from https://newsinhealth.nih.gov/2016/03/understanding-anxiety-disorders

Rubinstein, B. L. N. (2007, May 14). How to Choose the Best Therapist or Counselor for You. Retrieved February 27, 2021, from https://www.goodtherapy.org/blog/how-to-find-a-therapist/

Signs You Are Healing From Anxiety and Depression. (2018, August 23). Retrieved February 27, 2021, from https://www.bayviewrecovery.com/rehab-blog/signs-you-are-healing-from-anxiety-and-depression/

www.ingramcontent.com/pod-product-compliance
Lightning Source LLC
Chambersburg PA
CBHW030244030426
42336CB00009B/255